MEDICAL CANNABIS

CLINICAL PRACTICE

To my "favourite boss" as per your request

Sally

HEALTH AND HUMAN DEVELOPMENT

JOAV MERRICK - SERIES EDITOR

NATIONAL INSTITUTE OF CHILD HEALTH
AND HUMAN DEVELOPMENT,
MINISTRY OF SOCIAL AFFAIRS, JERUSALEM

Cannabis: Medical Aspects
Blair Henry, Arnav Agarwal,
Edward Chow, Hatim A Omar,
and Joav Merrick (Editors)
2017. ISBN: 978-1-53610-510-0
(Hardcover)
2017. ISBN: 978-1-53610-522-3
(eBook)

Alternative Medicine Research
Yearbook 2016
Joav Merrick (Editor)
2017. ISBN: 978-1-53610-972-6
(Hardcover)
2017. ISBN: 978-1-53611-000-5
(eBook)

Palliative Care: Psychosocial
and Ethical Considerations
Blair Henry, Arnav Agarwal,
Edward Chow, and Joav Merrick
(Editors)
2017. ISBN: 978-1-53610-607-7
(Hardcover)
2017. ISBN: 978-1-53610-611-4
(eBook)

Public Health Yearbook 2016
Joav Merrick (Editor)
2017. ISBN: 978-1-53610-947-4
(Hardcover)
2017. ISBN: 978-1-53610-956-6
(eBook)

Oncology: The Promising Future
of Biomarkers
Anthony Furfari,
George S Charames,
Rachel McDonald,
Leigha Rowbottom,
Azar Azad, Stephanie Chan,
Bo Angela Wan, Ronald Chow,
Carlo DeAngelis, Pearl Zaki,
Edward Chow and Joav Merrick
(Editors)
2017. ISBN: 978-1-53610-608-4
(Hardcover)
2017. ISBN: 978-1-53610-610-7
(eBook)

Pain Management Yearbook 2016
Joav Merrick (Editor)
2017. ISBN: 978-1-53610-949-8
(Hardcover)
2017. ISBN: 978-1-53610-959-7
(eBook)

Medical Cannabis:
Clinical Practice
Shannon O'Hearn, Alexia Blake,
Bo Angela Wan, Stephanie Chan,
Edward Chow and Joav Merrick
(Editors)
2017. ISBN: 978-1-53611-907-7
(Softcover)
2017. ISBN: 978-1-53611-927-5
(eBook)

Cancer: Treatment, Decision
Making and Quality of Life
Breanne Lechner, Ronald Chow,
Natalie Pulenzas, Marko Popovic,
Na Zhang, Xiaojing Zhang,
Edward Chow, and Joav Merrick
(Editors)
2016. ISBN: 978-1-63483-863-4
(Hardcover)
2015. ISBN: 978-1-63483-882-5
(eBook)

Cancer: Bone Metastases, CNS
Metastases and Pathological
Fractures
Breanne Lechner, Ronald Chow,
Natalie Pulenzas, Marko Popovic,
Na Zhang, Xiaojing Zhang,
Edward Chow, and Joav Merrick
(Editors)
2016. ISBN: 978-1-63483-949-5
(Hardcover)
2015. ISBN: 978-1-63483-960-0
(eBook)

Cancer: Spinal Cord, Lung,
Breast, Cervical, Prostate, Head
and Neck Cancer
Breanne Lechner, Ronald Chow,
Natalie Pulenzas, Marko Popovic,
Na Zhang, Xiaojing Zhang,
Edward Chow and Joav Merrick
(Editors)
2016. ISBN: 978-1-63483-904-4
(Hardcover)
2015. ISBN: 978-1-63483-911-2
(eBook)

Cancer: Survival, Quality of Life
and Ethical Implications
Breanne Lechner, Ronald Chow,
Natalie Pulenzas, Marko Popovic,
Na Zhang, Xiaojing Zhang,
Edward Chow and Joav Merrick
(Editors)
2016. ISBN: 978-1-63483-905-1
(Hardcover)
2015. ISBN: 978-1-63483-912-9
(eBook)

Cancer: Pain and Symptom
Management
Breanne Lechner, Ronald Chow,
Natalie Pulenzas, Marko Popovic,
Na Zhang, Xiaojing Zhang,
Edward Chow, and Joav Merrick
(Editors)
2016. ISBN: 978-1-63483-905-1
(Hardcover)
2015. ISBN: 978-1-63483-881-8
(eBook)

Textbook on Evidence-Based
Holistic Mind-Body Medicine:
Holistic Practice of Traditional
Hippocratic Medicine
Søren Ventegodt and Joav Merrick
2013. ISBN: 978-1-62257-105-5
(Hardcover)
2012. ISBN: 978-1-62257-174-1
(eBook)

Textbook on Evidence-Based
Holistic Mind-Body Medicine:
Healing the Mind in Traditional
Hippocratic Medicine
Søren Ventegodt and Joav Merrick
2013. ISBN: 978-1-62257-112-3
(Hardcover)
2012. ISBN: 978-1-62257-175-8
(eBook)

Textbook on Evidence-Based
Holistic Mind-Body Medicine:
Sexology and Traditional
Hippocratic Medicine
Søren Ventegodt and Joav Merrick
2013. ISBN: 978-1-62257-130-7
(Hardcover)
2012. ISBN: 978-1-62257-176-5
(eBook)

Conceptualizing Behavior in
Health and Social Research:
A Practical Guide to Data
Analysis
*Said Shahtahmasebi
and Damon Berridge*
2013. ISBN: 978-1-60876-383-2

Pediatric and Adolescent
Sexuality and Gynecology:
Principles for the Primary
Care Clinician
*Hatim A Omar,
Donald E Greydanus,
Artemis K Tsitsika, Dilip R Patel
and Joav Merrick (Editors)*
2013. ISBN: 978-1-60876-735-9
(Softcover)

Human Development: Biology
from a Holistic Point of View
*Søren Ventegodt,
Tyge Dahl Hermansen
and Joav Merrick*
2013. ISBN: 978-1-61470-441-6
(Hardcover)
2011. ISBN: 978-1-61470-541-3
(eBook)

Human Immunodeficiency Virus (HIV) Research: Social Science Aspects
Hugh Klein and Joav Merrick (Editors)
2012. ISBN: 978-1-62081-293-8 (Hardcover)
2012. ISBN: 978-1-62081-346-1 (eBook)

AIDS and Tuberculosis: Public Health Aspects
Daniel Chemtob and Joav Merrick (Editors)
2012. ISBN: 978-1-62081-382-9 (Softcover)
2012. ISBN: 978-1-62081-406-2 (eBook)

Public Health Yearbook 2011
Joav Merrick (Editor)
2012. ISBN: 978-1-62081-433-8 (Hardcover)
2012. ISBN: 978-1-62081-434-5 (eBook)

Alternative Medicine Research Yearbook 2011
Joav Merrick (Editor)
2012. ISBN: 978-1-62081-476-5 (Hardcover)
2012. ISBN: 978-1-62081-477-2 (eBook)

Building Community Capacity: Skills and Principles
Rosemary M Caron and Joav Merrick (Editors)
2012. ISBN: 978-1-61209-331-4 (Hardcover)
2012. ISBN: 978-1-62257-238-0 (eBook)

Textbook on Evidence-Based Holistic Mind-Body Medicine: Basic Principles of Healing in Traditional Hippocratic Medicine
Søren Ventegodt and Joav Merrick
2012. ISBN: 978-1-62257-094-2 (Hardcover)
2012. ISBN: 978-1-62257-172-7 (eBook)

Textbook on Evidence-Based Holistic Mind-Body Medicine: Basic Philosophy and Ethics of Traditional Hippocratic Medicine
Søren Ventegodt and Joav Merrick
2012. ISBN: 978-1-62257-052-2 (Hardcover)
2013. ISBN: 978-1-62257-707-1 (eBook)

**Textbook on Evidence-Based
Holistic Mind-Body Medicine:
Research, Philosophy, Economy
and Politics of Traditional
Hippocratic Medicine**
Søren Ventegodt and Joav Merrick
2012. ISBN: 978-1-62257-140-6
(Hardcover)
2012. ISBN: 978-1-62257-171-0
(eBook)

Behavioral Pediatrics, 3rd Edition
*Donald E Greydanus, Dilip R Patel,
Helen D Pratt and
Joseph L Calles, Jr (Editors)*
2011. ISBN: 978-1-60692-702-1
(Hardcover)
2009. ISBN: 978-1-60876-630-7
(eBook)

**Rural Child Health:
International Aspects**
Erica Bell and Joav Merrick (Editors)
2011. ISBN: 978-1-60876-357-3
(Hardcover)
2011. ISBN: 978-1-61324-005-2
(eBook)

**Environment, Mood Disorders
and Suicide**
*Teodor T Postolache
and Joav Merrick (Editors)*
2011. ISBN: 978-1-61668-505-8
(Hardcover)
2011. ISBN: 978-1-62618-340-7
(eBook)

**International Aspects
of Child Abuse and Neglect**
*Howard Dubowitz and Joav Merrick
(Editors)*
2011. ISBN: 978-1-60876-703-8
(Hardcover)
2010. ISBN: 978-1-61122-049-0
(Softcover)
2010. ISBN: 978-1-61122-403-0
(eBook)

**Positive Youth Development:
Evaluation and Future
Directions in a Chinese Context**
*Daniel TL Shek, Hing Keung Ma
and Joav Merrick (Editors)*
2011. ISBN: 978-1-60876-830-1
(Hardcover)
2011. ISBN: 978-1-62100-175-1
(Softcover)
2010. ISBN: 978-1-61209-091-7
(eBook)

**Understanding Eating Disorders:
Integrating Culture,
Psychology and Biology**
*Yael Latzer, Joav Merrick
and Daniel Stein (Editors)*
2011. ISBN: 978-1-61728-298-0
(Hardcover)
2011. ISBN: 978-1-61470-976-3
(Softcover)
2011. ISBN: 978-1-61942-054-0
(eBook)

Climate Change and Rural
Child Health
*Erica Bell, Bastian M Seidel
and Joav Merrick (Editors)*
2011. ISBN: 978-1-61122-640-9
(Hardcover)
2011. ISBN: 978-1-61209-014-6
(eBook)

Rural Medical Education:
Practical Strategies
*Erica Bell, Craig Zimitat
and Joav Merrick (Editors)*
2011. ISBN: 978-1-61122-649-2
(Hardcover)
2011. ISBN: 978-1-61209-476-2
(eBook)

Advances in Environmental
Health Effects of Toxigenic Mold
and Mycotoxins
Ebere Cyril Anyanwu
2011. ISBN: 978-1-60741-953-2

Public Health Yearbook 2009
Joav Merrick (Editor)
2011. ISBN: 978-1-61668-911-7
(Hardcover)
2011. ISBN: 978-1-62417-365-3
(eBook)

Child Health and Human
Development Yearbook 2009
Joav Merrick (Editor)
2011. ISBN: 978-1-61668-912-4

Alternative Medicine
Yearbook 2009
Joav Merrick (Editor)
2011. ISBN: 978-1-61668-910-0
(Hardcover)
2011. ISBN: 978-1-62081-710-0
(eBook)

The Dance of Sleeping and Eating
among Adolescents:
Normal and Pathological
Perspectives
*Yael Latzer and Orna Tzischinsky
(Editors)*
2011. ISBN: 978-1-61209-710-7
(Hardcover)
2011. ISBN: 978-1-62417-366-0
(eBook)

Drug Abuse in Hong Kong:
Development and Evaluation
of a Prevention Program
*Daniel TL Shek, Rachel CF Sun
and Joav Merrick (Editors)*
2011. ISBN: 978-1-61324-491-3
(Hardcover)
2011. ISBN: 978-1-62257-232-8
(eBook)

Chance Action and Therapy:
The Playful Way of Changing
Uri Wernik
2010. ISBN: 978-1-60876-393-1
(Hardcover)
2011. ISBN: 978-1-61122-987-5
(Softcover)
2011. ISBN: 978-1-61209-874-6
(eBook)

Bone and Brain Metastases:
Advances in Research
and Treatment
*Arjun Sahgal, Edward Chow
and Joav Merrick (Editors)*
2010. ISBN: 978-1-61668-365-8
(Hardcover)
2010. ISBN: 978-1-61728-085-6
(eBook)

Poverty and Children:
A Public Health Concern
*Alexis Lieberman and Joav Merrick
(Editors)*
2009. ISBN: 978-1-60741-140-6
(Hardcover)
2009. ISBN: 978-1-61470-601-4
(eBook)

Living on the Edge:
The Mythical, Spiritual,
and Philosophical Roots
of Social Marginality
Joseph Goodbread
2009. ISBN: 978-1-60741-162-8
(Hardcover)
2013. ISBN: 978-1-61122-986-8
(Softcover)
2011. ISBN: 978-1-61470-192-7
(eBook)

Alcohol-Related Cognitive
Disorders: Research and
Clinical Perspectives
*Leo Sher, Isack Kandel
and Joav Merrick (Editors)*
2009. ISBN: 978-1-60741-730-9
(Hardcover)
2009. ISBN: 978-1-60876-623-9
(eBook)

Children and Pain
*Patricia Schofield and Joav Merrick
(Editors)*
2009. ISBN: 978-1-60876-020-6
(Hardcover)
2009. ISBN: 978-1-61728-183-9
(eBook)

HEALTH AND HUMAN DEVELOPMENT

MEDICAL CANNABIS

CLINICAL PRACTICE

SHANNON O'HEARN

ALEXIA BLAKE

BO ANGELA WAN

STEPHANIE CHAN

EDWARD CHOW

AND

JOAV MERRICK

EDITORS

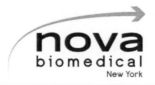

nova
biomedical
New York

NOTICE TO THE READER

Library of Congress Cataloging-in-Publication Data

ISBN: 978-1-53611-907-7

Published by Nova Science Publishers, Inc. † New York

CONTENTS

INTRODUCTION

In: Medical Cannabis ISBN: 978-1-53611-907-7
Editors: S. O'Hearn, A. Blake et al. © 2017 Nova Science Publishers, Inc.

Chapter 1

HOW CAN WE ADVANCE THE ADOPTION OF MEDICAL CANNABIS INTO CLINICAL PRACTICE?

Bo Angela Wan[1,], MPhil, Leila Malek[1], BSc (Hons),
Patrick Diaz[1], PhD(C), Carlo DeAngelis[1], PharmD,
Edward Chow[1], MBBS
and Joav Merrick[2-6], MD, MMedSc, DMSc*
[1]Odette Cancer Centre, Sunnybrook Health Sciences Centre,
University of Toronto, Toronto, Ontario, Canada
[2]National Institute of Child Health and Human Development, Jerusalem, Israel
[3]Division of Pediatrics, Hadassah Hebrew University Medical Center,
Mt Scopus Campus, Jerusalem, Israel
[4]Kentucky Children's Hospital, University of Kentucky School of Medicine,
Lexington, Kentucky, United States of America
[5]Center for Healthy Development, School of Public Health,
Georgia State University, Atlanta, United States of America
[6]Office of the Medical Director, Health Services,
Division for Intellectual and Developmental Disabilities
Ministry of Social Affairs and Social Services, Jerusalem, Israel

* Correspondence: Ms Bo Angela Wan, care of Professor Edward Chow, Department of Radiation Oncology, Odette Cancer Centre, Sunnybrook Health Sciences Centre, 2075 Bayview Avenue, Toronto ON, Canada. E-mail: Edward.Chow@sunnybrook.ca.

Medical cannabis is emerging as an effective treatment option for the management of a variety of common chronic conditions and symptoms, but a lack of scientific evidence demonstrating its efficacy for treating specific indications is hindering the widespread clinical adoption of medical cannabis. Between January 2015 and December 2016, patients who were prescribed medical cannabis in Canada from a single licensed medical cannabis provider were invited to complete an online survey approximately 15-25 minutes in length that assessed baseline demographics. Patients who completed the baseline survey were subsequently invited to complete follow-up surveys at 4 months and 10-months after completion of the initial survey. The results are described in this book and we hope the information will further facilitate the use of medical cannabis for the benefit of various populations in need.

INTRODUCTION

Medical cannabis is emerging as an effective treatment option for the management of a variety of symptoms and conditions, including pain, nausea, vomiting, post-traumatic stress disorder (PTSD), and insomnia (1–3). However, the lack of quality scientific evidence validating its efficacy for these indications has created barriers to its widespread adoption into regular clinical practice. Advancing the adoption of medical cannabis in the clinical setting can be achieved in three steps. First, extensive clinical research is required to further our understanding of the intricate interactions between cannabinoids, terpenes, and the endocannabinoid system. Secondly, patient reported outcomes must also be collected as a means of validating clinical research findings, and to gain valuable insight on the patient experience with medical cannabis treatment. Finally, this information will enable the development of highly efficacious, indication-specific cannabis products that, following clinical validation, will offer physicians and patients different dosage forms with specific therapeutic properties, thereby furthering the clinical utility of medical cannabis.

THE NEED TO CONDUCT HIGH QUALITY
SCIENTIFIC RESEARCH

Current evidence supporting the use of medical cannabis for the treatment of various symptoms and conditions is largely anecdotal or case-study based (2). To establish the efficacy of medical cannabis for its many indications, it is important that its safety and efficacy are further investigated in later stage controlled clinical trials. This includes phase II clinical trials assessing the efficacy and safety of medical cannabis for specific patient populations, followed by randomized phase III clinical trials to validate efficacy in larger patient populations. Efficacy studies should be strain-specific, with the intention of learning more about the physiological effects of specific cannabinoids and terpenes, their interactions with each other, and with the endocannabinoid system. This is essential for learning more about the structure and function of the endocannabinoid system, and how cannabis can be delivered most effectively to precisely interact with different components of this system to achieve targeted and desired effects.

It is also important to compare the safety and efficacy of medical cannabis to current clinical alternatives. Additionally, the effects of long term use or co-administration with other drugs remain unclear and should be further investigated (4). The results of such studies will establish which conditions can benefit from treatment with medical cannabis, and if certain dosage formats and strains are more effective for treating certain conditions.

THE NEED TO COLLECT ACCURATE PATIENT
REPORTED OUTCOMES

Patient reported outcomes can be a valuable tool for evaluating the efficacy of specific medical cannabis strains or products. However, it is important that this information is collected using non-biased and validated clinical tools to ensure that the captured data is objective, accurate and useful. Patient reported outcomes can validate clinical research findings related to the physiological effects and efficacy of specific strains. With this information, physicians will be able to prescribe specific strains to selectively treat certain symptoms or conditions, with confidence that the selected strain will be effective. The collection of patient outcomes should be performed systematically and take into account common confounding factors that exist in treatment routines, including the simultaneous use of more than one strain or product, and inconsistent dosage titrations. These factors are particularly important to consider since the dosing regimen may vary widely for patients using medical cannabis for different indications.

THE NEED TO PRODUCE A VARIETY OF EFFICACIOUS MEDICAL CANNABIS PRODUCTS

Medical cannabis is used to manage a variety of symptoms across numerous patient populations with different treatment needs (1–3). The variety of dosage forms available to patients should reflect these differences, so that the method of administration, pharmacokinetics, and clinical effects are appropriate for treating the symptom or condition in question. For instance, dosage forms developed for rapid absorption such as suppositories, sublingual tablets, and dried bud for inhalation may be better suited for treating breakthrough pain, or as delivery methods for patients with gastrointestinal issues or difficulty swallowing (5). Alternatively, topical products such as lotions and patches offer localized and targeted relief for patients suffering from arthritis and pain. Edibles or capsules with sustained-release action may be effective for patients with insomnia, anxiety, depression, or epilepsy, as these indications require sustained drug action (4).

However, such products must be subject to stringent validation in a controlled clinical setting to ensure that they are safe, suitable, and highly efficacious for specific conditions or patient groups. As more medical cannabis products become available to patients, it is also important to establish pharmacokinetic behavior and dose equivalencies between different dosage forms, including dried plant, cannabis oils, suppositories, topical creams, and tablets (4). Clinical research should focus on and encourage the clinical adoption of dosage forms in which concentrations of active ingredients can be specified and standardized, rather than dried cannabis administered by inhalation. This is because complete standardization of dried cannabis is near impossible to achieve, due to variation in cannabinoid and terpene composition among different plants (6). This framework would enable patients and healthcare professionals to make informed decisions when selecting cannabis products or switching between products with different methods of administration, allowing the treatment method to be tailored to the patient's needs while remaining consistently effective.

CONCLUSION

Medical cannabis is an emerging treatment option for the effective management of a variety of chronic conditions and symptoms that afflict a diverse patient population. However, adoption into regular clinical practice has been hindered due to a lack of scientific evidence demonstrating its efficacy for treating specific indications. Efficacy-based clinical trials and accurate patient reported outcomes will provide valuable insight into the therapeutic potential of medical cannabis, either as a primary or alternative treatment method. Additionally, this information can be used to develop highly efficacious cannabis products in different dosage forms that offer unique therapeutic benefits. This will allow doctors to prescribe medical cannabis with the confidence that the strain or dosage format recommended to their patients will be highly effective and safe, both in the long and short term.

REFERENCES

[1]   Borgelt LM, Franson KL, Nussbaum AM, Wang GS. The pharmacologic and clinical effects of medical cannabis. Pharmacotherapy 2013;33(2):195–209.

[2]   Hill KP. Medical marijuana for treatment of chronic pain and other medical and psychiatric problems. JAMA 2015;313(24):2474.

[3]   Whiting PF, Wolff RF, Deshpande S, Di Nisio M, Duffy S, Hernandez AV, et al. Cannabinoids for medical use. JAMA 2015;313(24):2456–73.

[4]   Grotenhermen   F.   Pharmacokinetics   and   pharmacodynamics   of cannabinoids. Clin Pharmacokinet 2003;42(4):327–60.

[5]   Ben Amar M. Cannabinoids in medicine: A review of their therapeutic potential. J Ethnopharmacol 2006;105(1–2):1–25.

[6]   Hill KP. Medical marijuana for treatment of chronic pain and other medical and psychiatric problems. JAMA 2015;313(24):2474.

SECTION ONE: MEDICAL CANNABIS

In: Medical Cannabis
ISBN: 978-1-53611-907-7
Editors: S. O'Hearn, A. Blake et al. © 2017 Nova Science Publishers, Inc.

Chapter 2

PATIENT CHARACTERISTICS FROM A MEDICAL CANNABIS PROVIDER

Bo Angela Wan[1], MPhil, Alexia Blake[2], MSc,
Stephanie Chan[1], BSc(C), Amiti Wolt[2], BA,
Pearl Zaki[1], BSc(C), Liying Zhang[1], PhD,
Marissa Slaven[3], MD, Erynn Shaw[3], MD,
Carlo DeAngelis[1], PharmD, Henry Lam[1], MLS,
Vithusha Ganesh[1], BSc(C), Leila Malek[1], BSc(Hons),
Edward Chow[1], MBBS and Shannon O'Hearn[2,], MSc*

[1]Odette Cancer Centre, Sunnybrook Health Sciences Centre,
University of Toronto, Toronto, Ontario, Canada
[2]MedReleaf, Markham, Ontario, Canada
[3]Juravinski Cancer Centre, Hamilton Health Sciences,
Hamilton, Ontario, Canada

* Correspondence: Ms. Shannon O'Hearn MSc, Project Manager, Clinical Research, MedReleaf, Markham Industrial Park, Markham, Ontario, Canada. Email: sohearn@medreleaf.com.

Medical cannabis has been prescribed by physicians to treat a variety of symptoms including pain, nausea and vomiting, anxiety, depression, and sleep disorders in patients with severe or chronic illnesses. This chapter presents the baseline demographics and characteristics of patients using medical cannabis in Canada. Patients were invited to complete a voluntary online survey after registering with a single medical cannabis provider. The survey included questions on demographics, medical history, current medical conditions and symptoms, and their corresponding severities. A total of 2,753 patients completed the survey (average age of 43.0 years old, SD=13.7). Patients were predominantly male (68.4%, n=1,882) and Caucasian (80.3%, n=2,089). Most patients were employed (49.4%, n=1133), while 18.7% (n=428) were retired, and 3.9% (n=89) were students. Of the surveyed patients, 25.1% (n=580) smoked tobacco cigarettes, and 74.9% (n=1782) reported having previous experience with cannabis. The most frequently reported conditions were anxiety disorder (31.7%, n=723), depression (31.6%, n=729), pain (29.5%, n=681), and sleep disorder (25.5%, n=589). The most frequently reported symptoms included pain (73.0%, n=2011), anxiety (72.6%, n=1998), and sleep problems (69.8%, n=1922). These findings are consistent with results from other North American studies, suggesting their generalizability in defining patient populations that may benefit from medical cannabis use. Understanding patient characteristics will be useful in informing the design of future clinical research initiatives and identifying the needs of patients using medical cannabis.

INTRODUCTION

The plant species *Cannabis sativa* has long been a part of human history and medicine; for example, it has been used in China due to its range of psychoactive and physiological effects for at least 5000 years (1). Cannabis contains a complex combination of active compounds with varying pharmacodynamics and pharmacologic properties (2–4). The most well-known of these compounds is delta-9-tetrahydrocannabinol (THC), which is also the major psychoactive component in cannabis (5). THC belongs to a group of compounds known as cannabinoids, of which over 100 distinct structural types have been identified (3). These compounds are structurally similar to endogenous cannabinoids such as the euphoriant neurotransmitter anandamide, which are a part of the mammalian endocannabinoid system (6). In humans, cannabinoids have been found to activate CB-1 and CB-2 receptors of this system. These receptors are found in neurons of the central and peripheral nervous systems, and their activation leads to a wide range of effects including modulation of pain, appetite, mood, and memory (4, 7, 8).

Cannabis can be used for a variety of therapeutic applications. A systematic meta-analysis conducted by Amar (1) reviewed the findings of 72 controlled studies examining the effects of medical cannabis across 10 different pathologies or symptoms (1). These included nausea and vomiting associated with chemotherapy, loss of appetite, pain, multiple sclerosis, spinal cord injuries, Tourette's syndrome, epilepsy, glaucoma, Parkinson's disease, and dystonia. Nine of the 14 studies assessing acute and chronic pain found a significant reduction in dose of opioids or other pain medications following cannabis use. The most recent of these studies was conducted by Berman et al, which investigated 48 patients with neuropathic pain and found a statistically significant reduction in pain and improvement in sleep after the administration of THC (9). This suggests that medical cannabis may be a safer and more effective alternative to opioid analgesics without the risk of addiction-associated with opioid use.

Medical cannabis has emerged as a potential alternative or concomitant treatment option for a variety of indications. The growing number of medical cannabis patients has drawn attention to the need to better understand the physiological mechanisms behind its effects, and the characteristics of populations that may benefit from its use. However, there is a lack of data assessing the demographic and medical characteristics of medical cannabis users. The purpose of the present study was to assess the characteristics of medical cannabis patients with the intention of understanding their medical needs and how cannabis may be used to alleviate their underlying medical conditions and associated symptoms. This knowledge will inform the design of future clinical research initiatives and contribute to the incorporation of medical cannabis into standard clinical practice.

OUR STUDY

Between January 2015 and December 2016, patients who were prescribed medical cannabis in Canada from a single licensed medical cannabis provider were invited to complete an online survey approximately 15-25 minutes in length that assessed baseline demographics. Patients who completed the baseline survey were subsequently invited to complete follow-up (FU) surveys at 4 months and 10-months after completion of the initial survey.

The survey was designed based on scientific literature with direction from scientists and healthcare professionals with experience prescribing medical cannabis for patient care. Pain was assessed on a scale of 1-10, which was derived from the numerical rating scale, a common validated method of reporting chronic pain (10–12). Assessment of overall quality of life (QOL) was based on the commonly used and validated Quality of Life Scale (13, 14).

The dynamic survey contained a bank of over 100 questions, from which a customized selection was given to patients based on their responses to previous survey questions. For example, patients who responded "no" to "have you ever smoked cigarettes?" were not asked to answer "how many cigarettes did you smoke?" Patients were given the option to skip questions they did not want to answer. In certain questions, patients were also given the option to select "prefer not to answer," or "other" and input a specific response. As each patient completed a customized survey that assessed only relevant attributes in detail, each question received a different number of responses.

The baseline survey assessed patient demographics and medical information. Demographic information collected included age, sex, ethnicity, smoking status, previous experience with cannabis, and employment status. Patients were asked to select any diagnosed conditions from a list of 46 conditions, and were prompted with FU questions regarding specific aspects of their condition. Patients were also asked to select present symptoms from a list of 39 symptoms and rate the severity of each symptom as "mild," "moderate," or "severe." Patients were asked to score severity of pain on a scale of 1-10, where 1 represented dull pain and 10 represented severe pain. Patients were asked to rate their ability to perform activities of daily living (ADLs) from very capable, to somewhat capable, somewhat incapable, very incapable, or don't know. Moreover, patients were asked about their experiences of sleep, appetite, concentration, bowel activity, and sexual function by selecting from severe difficulty, moderate difficulty, no difficulty, good, or very good. Patients were also asked about any difficulties with mobility, and ability to dress and shower independently through selecting from severe, moderate, minimal, or no difficulty.

Patients who selected "other" as an answer to any question were asked to specify, and their responses were categorized into existing options where appropriate. Data was summarized with statistical parameters of median, mean, range, standard deviation (SD), and percentage of total when appropriate.

FINDINGS

A total of 2,753 patients identified their age and sex (see Table 1). Patient ages ranged from 2-91 years old, with the average age being 43.0 years old (SD=13.7 years). A larger percentage (68.4%, n=1,882) of the surveyed population was male.

Table 2 summarizes the lifestyle demographics of the surveyed patients. Of 2,314 patients who responded to the question "Do you smoke tobacco cigarettes?," 25.1% (n=580) responded "yes." FU questions showed that individuals smoked anywhere from one cigarette/day to over 60 cigarettes/day, with a median of 12 cigarettes/day. The duration of tobacco cigarette smoking ranged from one year to 30 years, with the median number of years ranging between 20-30.

Of the 2,319 patients who provided information about previous experience with cannabis, most responders reported that they had previous experience (76.8%, n=1,782), while 15.8% (n=366) had not used cannabis before (see Table 2). The remaining patients preferred not to answer this question (7.4%, n=171).

Table 1. Patient age distribution by sex

	Male	Female
Age (Years)	n (%)	n (%)
0-19	20 (0.7%)	11 (0.4%)
20-29	303 (11%)	96 (3.5%)
30-39	543 (19.7%)	196 (7.1%)
40-49	405 (14.7%)	184 (6.7%)
50-59	380 (13.8%)	244 (8.9%)
60-69	182 (6.6%)	105 (3.8%)
70-79	41 (1.5%)	22 (0.8%)
80-89	7 (0.3%)	13 (0.5%)
90-99	1 (0.04%)	0 (0%)
Total	1882 (68.4%)	871 (31.6%)
Overall Total	2753	
Average (SD)	43.0 (13.7)	
Median (Range)	45 (1, 92)	

SD: Standard deviation.

Of the 2,293 patients who specified their employment status, 34.5% (n=791) were employed full-time, while 18.7% (n=428) were retired, 10.9% (n=236) were not employed and not looking for work, 9.7% (n=222) were self-employed, and 3.9% (n=89) were students.

A total of 2,602 patients indicated their ethnicity, with the majority of patients identifying as "Caucasian" (80.3%, n=2089), followed by "Native Canadian" (4.8%, n=126), "Asian" (3.5%, n=90), "Black/African American/African" (1.7%, n=43), and "Spanish/Hispanic/Latino" (0.9%, n=23) (see Table 3). A single individual identified as being "Pacific Islander" (0.04%). As several individuals indicated more than one race, these responses were collectively grouped under "Mixed race," which made up 1.5% of all responses (n=38).

Table 2. Patient lifestyle demographics

	n (%)
Smoking status	
Smoker	580 (25.1%)
Non-smoker	1734 (74.9%)
Total responses	2314
Experience with Cannabis	
Yes	1782 (76.8%)
No	366 (15.8%)
Prefer not to answer	171 (7.4%)
Total responses	2319
Employment status	
Employed Full-Time	791 (34.5%)
Employed Part-Time	120 (5.2%)
Self-Employed	222 (9.7%)
Not employed, but looking for work	129 (5.6%)
Not employed, and not looking for work	236 (10.3%)
Homemaker	88 (3.8%)
Retired	428 (18.7%)
Student	89 (3.9%)
Prefer Not to Answer	190 (8.3%)
Total Responses	2293

Table 3. Patient ethnicities

Ethnicity	n (%)	Census Canada 2011 (%)
White/Caucasian	2089 (80.3%)	67.6%
Native Canadian	126 (4.8%)	4.3%
Spanish/Hispanic/Latino	23 (0.9%)	1.2%
Black/African American/African	43 (1.7%)	2.9%
Asian/Middle Eastern/South Asian	90 (3.5%)	14.2%
Pacific Islander	1 (0.04%)	N/A
Mixed race	38 (1.5%)	0.5%
Prefer Not to Answer	164 (6.3%)	N/A
Other	28 (1.1%)	N/A
Total Responses	2602	

Patients were asked to specify their diagnosed condition(s) from a list of 46 conditions, or to indicate any additional conditions that had not been specified. Responses were obtained from 2,307 patients, with the twenty most commonly diagnosed conditions listed in Table 4. The most highly reported conditions were anxiety disorder (31.7%, n=732), followed closely by depression (31.6%, n=729) and pain (29.5%, n=681). Additional common conditions included sleep disorder (25.5%, n=589) and post-traumatic stress disorder PTSD (21.8%, n=502).

Table 4. Patient medical conditions

Medical Condition	n (%)
Anxiety Disorder	732 (31.7%)
Depression	729 (31.6%)
Pain	681 (29.5%)
Sleep disorder	589 (25.5%)
PTSD	502 (21.8%)
Migraines	336 (14.6%)
Degenerative Disc Disease	278 (12.1%)
Irritable bowel syndrome	247 (10.7%)
Fibromyalgia	214 (9.3%)
Spinal Disk Herniation	194 (8.4%)
ADHD	169 (7.3%)
Cancer	142 (6.2%)
Restless Leg Syndrome	137 (5.9%)
Asthma	128 (5.5%)
GERD	120 (5.2%)
Hypertension	116 (5.0%)
Diabetes	96 (4.2%)
Obsessive Compulsive Disorder	74 (3.2%)
Bipolar	71 (3.1%)
Diverticulitis	50 (2.2%)
Total Responses	2307

PTSD: Post-traumatic stress disorder
ADHD: Attention deficit hyperactivity disorder
GERD: Gastroesophageal reflux disease

Table 5. Patient symptoms and distribution of symptom severities

Symptom	Total, n (%)	Mild, n (%)	Moderate, n (%)	Severe, n (%)
Pain	2011 (73%)	192 (9.5%)	815 (40.5%)	1004 (49.9%)
Anxiety	1998 (72.6%)	531 (26.6%)	993 (49.7%)	474 (23.7%)
Sleep problems	1922 (69.8%)	382 (19.9%)	890 (46.3%)	650 (33.8%)
Depression	1632 (59.3%)	536 (32.8%)	739 (45.3%)	357 (21.9%)
Insomnia	1529 (55.5%)	339 (22.2%)	698 (45.7%)	492 (32.2%)
Exhaustion	1386 (50.3%)	371 (26.8%)	662 (47.8%)	353 (25.5%)
Headache	1322 (48%)	508 (38.4%)	522 (39.5%)	292 (22.1%)
Digestion problems	1085 (39.4%)	406 (37.4%)	500 (46.1%)	179 (16.5%)
Limited mobility	1082 (39.3%)	339 (31.3%)	495 (45.7%)	248 (22.9%)
Constipation	978 (35.5%)	483 (49.4%)	356 (36.4%)	139 (14.2%)
Dry mouth	969 (35.2%)	457 (47.2%)	377 (38.9%)	135 (13.9%)
Weakness	956 (34.7%)	408 (42.7%)	424 (44.4%)	124 (13%)
Numbness	924 (33.6%)	380 (41.1%)	377 (40.8%)	167 (18.1%)
Drowsiness	893 (32.4%)	408 (45.7%)	386 (43.2%)	99 (11.1%)
Nausea	870 (31.6%)	441 (50.7%)	317 (36.4%)	112 (12.9%)
Dizziness	829 (30.1%)	510 (61.5%)	272 (32.8%)	47 (5.7%)
Burning sensation	823 (29.9%)	304 (36.9%)	331 (40.2%)	188 (22.8%)
Diarrhea	818 (29.7%)	408 (49.9%)	282 (34.5%)	128 (15.6%)
Spasms	809 (29.4%)	304 (37.6%)	363 (44.9%)	142 (17.6%)
Cognitive impairment	798 (29%)	387 (48.5%)	326 (40.9%)	85 (10.7%)
Total responses	2753			

Patients were presented with a list of 39 symptoms and asked to indicate which of these they currently experience. They were also asked to rate the severity of their symptoms as mild, moderate, or severe. Table 5 shows the twenty most commonly reported symptoms from 2753 patients. Pain was the most highly reported symptom (73.0%, n=2,011), followed by anxiety (72.6%, n=1,988), sleep problems (69.8%, n=1,922), depression (59.3%, n=1,632), insomnia (55.5%, n=1,529), and exhaustion (50.3%, n=1,368).

The distributions of symptom severities varied widely. The most frequently experienced symptoms of current cannabis patients were also most commonly reported as being severe rather than moderate or mild. For example, pain was the most frequently reported symptom, and out of the 2,011 patients who reported pain, 49.9% experienced severe pain (n=1,004). Sleep problems also commonly manifested as being severe, with 33.8% of the 1,922 patients with sleep problems reporting severe sleep problems (n=650).

DISCUSSION

When compared to the racial distribution of the Canadian population from the most national census, Census Canada 2011, the racial distribution of cannabis patients in this study showed that "White/Caucasian," "Native Canadian," and "Mixed" races were more highly represented (15) (see Table 3). "Spanish/Hispanic/Latino," "Black/African American," and "Asian" ethnicities were less represented in the medical cannabis patient population when compared to the general Canadian population.

The present study analyzing the baseline demographics of patients using medical cannabis is the largest study of this nature conducted to date in Canada. A smaller study conducted in Canada by Walsh et al. assessed 702 medical cannabis users recruited across the country, and 77 local medical cannabis users recruited from a cannabis dispensary in British Columbia (16). Similar to the present study, an adaptive online questionnaire was used to collect information pertaining to patient demographics and relevant medical conditions or symptoms. In this study, Walsh et al. found the most commonly reported symptoms and conditions for which patients were using medical cannabis were sleep disorders (85%), pain (82%), anxiety (79%), and depression (67%) (see Table 4).

In the United States, Reinarman et al. studied a sample of 1,746 patients from medical evaluation clinics in California, and found that users were predominantly Caucasian and male (17). The most common conditions approved by physicians for cannabis use included pain (30.6%), sleep disorders (15.7%), and anxiety or depression (13.0%) (17). A study involving 347 patients recruited from four medical cannabis dispensaries in Arizona was conducted by Trout et al. (18). Although this study did not assess patient demographics, it reported existing patient conditions and symptoms (18). The authors showed that a large proportion of patients suffered from chronic pain (86.6%), anxiety (49.3%), stress (44.7%), and insomnia (39.5%) (18). In the United Kingdom, a study by Ware et al. on 2,969 cannabis patients found that medical cannabis users were most commonly afflicted with chronic pain (25%), depression (22%), and multiple sclerosis (22%) (19). They also found that medical cannabis use was more common among younger males. The North American findings on commonly reported patient symptoms were similar to those reported in the present study, namely pain, anxiety, sleep problems, and depression. However, they slightly differed from that of the UK where multiple sclerosis was one of the common uses for medical cannabis. Since the prevalence of multiple sclerosis is similar in UK and Canada, it is unlikely that this represents a true demographic difference (20). This difference is likely due to regulations regarding the indications for which a physician can prescribe medical cannabis, highlighting the importance of policy on impacting patient access to treatment. Similar to the previously mentioned studies, a majority of patients in the present study were male.

The commonalities between medical cannabis users across a variety of populations from these studies, covering Canada, USA, and UK, suggest that individuals likely to benefit from medical cannabis have a shared set of symptoms and characteristics including anxiety, depression, stress, and pain. Therefore, these results are applicable to a broad patient population and may be able to predict if cannabis is a suitable treatment option for patients based on their symptoms.

One limitation to this study is that the survey was designed as a voluntary online survey in which results were self-reported, and patients were given the option to not answer certain questions. Therefore, not all patients answered the same questions and the received responses may be influenced by selection and recall bias.

CONCLUSION

Demographic and medical characteristics of patients who were prescribed medical cannabis and participated in this study were consistent with previously published data in North America. The present Canadian study showed that cannabis patients suffered from a variety of conditions and symptoms, the most common of which were anxiety, depression, and pain. Additionally, sleep disorders and PTSD were prevalent among the surveyed patient population. The demographic characteristics of cannabis users were diverse, but patients were predominantly Caucasian males, most of whom were employed. Understanding the demographic profile of patients using medical cannabis may assist physicians in identifying patients who are likely to benefit from medical cannabis. Additionally, understanding patient population demographics is essential for guiding future clinical research initiatives so that research is targeted towards patient populations who are suitable candidates for medical cannabis treatment.

ACKNOWLEDGMENT

We thank the generous support of Bratty Family Fund, Michael and Karyn Goldstein Cancer Research Fund, Joey and Mary Furfari Cancer Research Fund, Pulenzas Cancer Research Fund, Joseph and Silvana Melara Cancer Research Fund, and Ofelia Cancer Research Fund. This study was conducted in collaboration with MedReleaf.

REFERENCES

[1]   Ben Amar M. Cannabinoids in medicine: A review of their therapeutic potential. J Ethnopharmacol 2006;105(1–2):1–25.
[2]   Grotenhermen F. The cannabinoid system-a brief review. J Ind Hemp 2004;9(2):87–92.

[3]   ElSohly MA, Slade D. Chemical constituents of marijuana: The complex mixture of natural cannabinoids. Life Sci 2005;78(5):539–48.

[4]   F. G. Clinical pharmacodynamics of cannabinoids. J Cannabis Ther 2004;4(1):29–78.

[5]   Manzanares J, Julian MD, Carrascosa A. Role of the cannabinoid system in pain control and therapeutic implications for the management of acute and chronic pain episodes. Curr Neuropharmacol 2006;4:239–57.

[6]   Huang W-J, Chen W-W, Zhang X. Endocannabinoid system: Role in depression, reward and pain control (Review). Mol Med Rep 2016;14:2899–903.

[7]   Fraser GA. The use of a synthetic cannabinoid in the management of treatment-resistant nightmares in posttraumatic stress disorder (PTSD). CNS Neurosci Ther 2009;15(1):84–8.

[8]   Hazekamp A, Grotenhermen F. Review on clinical studies with cannabis and cannabinoids 2005-2009. Cannainoids 2010;5:1–21.

[9]   Berman JS, Symonds C, Birch R. Efficacy of two cannabis based medicinal extracts for relief of central neuropathic pain from brachial plexus avulsion: Results of a randomised controlled trial. Pain 2004;112(3):299–306.

[10]   Krebs EE, Carey TS, Weinberger M. Accuracy of the pain numeric rating scale as a screening test in primary care. J Gen Intern Med 2007;22(10):1453–8.

[11]   Hawker GA, Mian S, Kendzerska T, French M. Measures of adult pain: Visual Analog Scale for Pain (VAS Pain), Numeric Rating Scale for Pain (NRS Pain), McGill Pain Questionnaire (MPQ), Short-Form McGill Pain Questionnaire (SF-MPQ), Chronic Pain Grade Scale (CPGS), Short Form-36 Bodily Pain Scale (SF-36 BPS), and Measure of Intermittent and Constant Osteoarthritis Pain (ICOAP). Arthritis Care Res 2011;63:240–52.

[12]   Farrar JT, Young JP, LaMoreaux L, Werth JL, Poole RM. Clinical importance of changes in chronic pain intensity measured on an 11-point numerical rating scale. Pain 2001;94(2):149–58.

[13]   Burckhardt CS, Anderson KL. The Quality of Life Scale (QOLS): reliability, validity, and utilization. Health Qual Life Outcomes 2003;1(1):60.

[14]   Fletcher A, Gore S, Jones D, Fitzpatrick R, Spiegelhalter D, Cox D. Quality of life measures in health care. II: Design, analysis, and interpretation. BMJ 1992;305(7):1145–8.

[15]   Statistics Canada. 211 Census: National Household Survey (NHS) Profile [internet]. 2013 [cited 2016 Nov 24]; Statistics Canada Catalogue no. 99-004-XWE. Available from: http://www12.statcan.gc.ca/nhs-enm/2011/dp-pd/prof/index.cfm?Lang=E.

[16]   Walsh Z, Callaway R, Belle-Isle L, Capler R, Kay R, Lucas P, et al. Cannabis for therapeutic purposes: Patient characteristics, access, and reasons for use. Int J Drug Policy 2013;24(6):511–6.

[17]   Reinarman C, Nunberg H, Lanthier F, Heddleston T. Who are medical marijuana patients? Population characteristics from nine California assessment clinics. J Psychoactive Drugs 2011;43(2):128–35.

[18]   Troutt WD, DiDonato MD. Medical cannabis in Arizona: Patient characteristics, perceptions, and impressions of medical cannabis legalization. J Psychoact Drugs Routledge; 2015;1072(May):1–8.

[19]   Ware MA, Adams H, Guy GW. The medicinal use of cannabis in the UK: Results of a nationwide survey. Int J Clin Pract 2005;59(3):291–5.

[20]   Browne P, Chandraratna D, Angood C, Tremlett H, Baker C, Taylor B V., et al. Atlas of Multiple Sclerosis 2013: A growing global problem with widespread inequity. Neurology 2014;83(11):1022–4.

In: Medical Cannabis   ISBN: 978-1-53611-907-7
Editors: S. O'Hearn, A. Blake et al. © 2017 Nova Science Publishers, Inc.

Chapter 3

SYMPTOM CLUSTERS IN PATIENT REPORTED OUTCOMES OF MEDICAL CANNABIS PATIENTS

Nicholas Lao[1], BMSc(C), Vithusha Ganesh[1], BSc(C),
Liying Zhang[1], PhD, Leah Drost[1], BSc(C),
Bo Angela Wan[1], MPhil, Alexia Blake[1,2], MSc,
Stephanie Chan[1], BSc(C), Amiti Wolt[2], BA,
Pearl Zaki[1], BSc(C), Marissa Slaven[3], MD,
Erynn Shaw[3], MD, Carlo DeAngelis[1], PharmD,
Henry Lam[1], MLS, Leila Malek[1], BSc(Hons),
Edward Chow[1], MBBS and Shannon O'Hearn[2,], MSc*

[1]Odette Cancer Centre, Sunnybrook Health Sciences Centre,
University of Toronto, Toronto, Ontario
[2]MedReleaf, Markham, Ontario
[3]Juravinski Cancer Centre, Hamilton Health Sciences,
Hamilton, Ontario, Canada

---

[*] Correspondence: Ms. Shannon O'Hearn MSc, Project Manager, Clinical Research, MedReleaf, Markham Industrial Park, Markham, Ontario, Canada. Email: sohearn@medreleaf.com.

Medical cannabis has been reported to be efficacious for managing symptoms associated with a variety of conditions, including cancer, anxiety, depression, and post-traumatic stress disorder. Symptom clusters have been identified in patients across a variety of conditions, and can be used by healthcare professionals to better manage patient quality of life. We aimed to identify baseline symptom clusters in patients registered with a Canadian medical cannabis provider. Principal component analysis (PCA) was performed using the PRINQUAL procedure to identify symptom clusters among the 10 most prevalent symptoms patients reported through a voluntary online survey administered after registration with their cannabis provider. The majority of respondents were male (69.2%), Caucasian (91.8%) and employed (50.9%). The average age of respondents was 46.5 years. Common conditions reported included chronic pain, sleep disorders, anxiety disorders, depression and post-traumatic stress disorder. Three clusters were identified using PCA, and displayed in biplots. Cluster 1 contained anxiety, depression, exhaustion, and sleep interference. Cluster 2 consisted of limited mobility, numbness, and pain. Cluster 3 included constipation, digestion problems, and headache. All clusters displayed good internal consistencies. Three symptom clusters were identified at baseline using PCA, with cluster 1 previously observed in cancer patients. The demographic and symptom profiles of respondents in the present study are also consistent with the limited literature that currently exists. Identifying symptom clusters in medical cannabis patients may allow physicians to make dosing and strain recommendations that will more effectively manage patients' overall condition(s) and commonly associated symptoms.

INTRODUCTION

Across various medical conditions, patients often present with multiple, interrelated symptoms, posing unique challenges to health care providers in terms of diagnosis and symptom management. Recent research on symptom clusters, defined as groups composed of a minimum of two concurrent symptoms, has helped mitigate this challenge (1). Symptom cluster research has been widely explored in the cancer patient population, as these patients often experience multiple symptoms which can be predictive of changes in patient function, treatment failures and post-therapeutic outcomes (2). Outside of cancer, symptom clusters have also been significantly reported in cardiovascular diseases such as angina, heart failure, acute coronary syndrome and stroke (3-5). Due to their clinical significance, it is important that symptom clusters in various patient populations are identified so that health care providers may facilitate effective therapies in symptom management.

Medical cannabis has garnered much interest of late for its therapeutic potential in the treatment of various symptoms and conditions (6). In their review article, Grotenhermen and Muller-Vahl commented on its use for only a few of these indications, including multiple sclerosis, nausea, chronic and neuropathic pain. Despite the increasing use of medical cannabis, there is little evidence regarding the demographic and symptom profile of current medical cannabis patients. A better understanding of symptom clusters in this population may help medical cannabis providers and clinicians strategically target concurrent symptoms with specific cannabis varieties. The purpose of the present study was to identify baseline symptom clusters in patients before beginning treatment with medical cannabis.

OUR PROJECT

Patients registered with a single Canadian licensed cannabis provider were invited to complete a voluntary online survey upon registration (baseline). The online survey was developed in consultation with various healthcare professionals knowledgeable on the topic of medical cannabis. The survey was dynamic, with answers to earlier questions determining subsequent questions asked. Patients were given the option to skip questions or choose more than one applicable answer for several questions. Information pertaining to patient demographics, current condition(s) and symptom(s), corresponding severity, and quality of life, was collected at baseline.

To examine whether any interrelationships existed among symptoms, a principal component analysis (PCA) for qualitative data was performed on the 10 most prevalent symptoms reported at baseline. The PRINQUAL procedure in Statistical Analysis Software (SAS version 9.4 for Windows) was used. The PCA transforms ordinal variables monotonically by scoring the ordered categories, so that the covariance matrix is optimized (7). The PRINQUAL procedure iterations produce a set of transformed variables. Each symptom's new scoring satisfies a set of constraints based on the original scoring of the symptom and the specified transformation type. The new set of scores is selected from the sets of possible scorings that do not violate the constraints so that the method criterion is locally optimized. The varimax rotation is an orthogonal rotation which results in uncorrelated components. Compared to other types of rotations, it tends to maximize the variance of a column of the factor pattern matrix.

The first principal component accounts for as much variability in the data as possible. The number of significant principal components was selected using a minimum Eigenvalue of 1.0. Each component explained more than 10% of the variance. The highest loading score predicted the assignment of individual symptoms to an independent factor. The internal consistency and reliability of the derived clusters were assessed with Cronbach's alpha. Robust relationships and correlations among symptoms were displayed with the bipolot graphic. The longer the length and closer the arrows were together, the higher the correlations between symptoms.

WHAT DID WE FIND?

Baseline responses collected between January 2015 and December 2016 from a total of 863 patients were included in the analysis. The majority of respondents were male (69.2%) and Caucasian (91.8%) (see Table 1). The average age of respondents was 46.5 years, and more than half were employed (50.9%).

The ten most prevalent symptoms reported at baseline were anxiety (79.5%), constipation (39.5%), depression (65.9%), digestion problems (43.7%), exhaustion (56.2%), headache (51.2%), sleep interference (82.8%), limited mobility (43.6%), numbness (38.2%) and pain (79.3%). Proportions of patient-reported symptom severity (none, mild, moderate, severe) is displayed in Table 2. Spearman correlations among the 10 symptoms are included in Table 3.

Table 1. Patient demographics (n=863)

Demographic	n (%)
Gender (Total n=859)	
Male	594 (69.2%)
Female	265 (30.8%)
Ethnicity (Total n=784)	
Caucasian	720 (91.8%)
Spanish/Hispanic/Latino	5 (0.6%)
Native Canadian	40 (5.1%)
Black/African American	9 (1.1%)
Asian	10 (1.3%)
Age (years) (Total n=832)	
19 – 29	71 (8.5%)
30 – 39	210 (25.2%)
40 – 49	185 (22.2%)
50 – 59	247 (29.7%)
60 – 69	98 (11.8%)
≥ 70	21 (2.5%)
Average (min, max)	46.5 (20, 80)
Previous experience with cannabis (Total n=802)	
Yes	681 (84.9%)
No	121 (15.1%)
Employment (Total n=776)	
Full-time	276 (35.6%)
Part-time	43 (5.5%)
Self-employed	76 (9.8%)
Unemployed	122 (15.7%)
Homemaker	32 (4.1%)
Retired	199 (25.6%)
Student	28 (3.6%)

Table 2. Descriptive analysis of symptom scores at baseline (n=863)

Symptoms (Total n=863)	n (%)
Anxiety	
None	177 (20.5%)
Mild	164 (19.0%)
Moderate	348 (40.3%)
Severe	174 (20.2%)
None	522 (60.5%)
Mild	172 (19.9%)
Moderate	119 (13.8%)

Table 2. (Continued)

Symptoms (Total n=863)	n (%)
Constipation	
Severe	50 (5.8%)
Depression	
None	294 (34.1%)
Mild	170 (19.7%)
Moderate	271 (31.4%)
Severe	128 (14.8%)
Digestion problems	
None	486 (56.3%)
Mild	129 (15%)
Moderate	181 (21%)
Severe	67 (7.8%)
Exhaustion	
None	378 (43.8%)
Mild	121 (14%)
Moderate	247 (28.6%)
Severe	117 (13.6%)
Headache	
None	421 (48.8%)
Mild	179 (20.7%)
Moderate	175 (20.3%)
Severe	88 (10.2%)
Sleep interference	
None	148 (17.2%)
Mild	135 (15.6%)
Moderate	335 (38.8%)
Severe	245 (28.4%)
Limited mobility	
None	487 (56.4%)
Mild	120 (13.9%)
Moderate	185 (21.4%)
Severe	71 (8.2%)
None	533 (61.8%)
Mild	133 (15.4%)
Moderate	143 (16.6%)
Severe	54 (6.3%)
Pain	
None	179 (20.7%)
Mild	60 (7%)
Moderate	277 (32.1%)
Severe	347 (40.2%)

Table 3. Spearman correlation among 10 symptoms with p-values (Total n=863)

Symptoms	Anxiety	Constipation	Depression	Digestion problems	Exhaustion	Headache	Sleep interference	Limited mobility	Numbness	Pain
Anxiety	1.00****									
Constipation	0.13***	1.00****								
Depression	0.59****	0.21****	1.00****							
Digestion problems	0.16****	0.48****	0.16****	1.00****						
Exhaustion	0.27****	0.37****	0.41****	0.33****	1.00****					
Headache	0.22****	0.30****	0.23****	0.28****	0.41****	1.00****				
Sleep interference	0.30****	0.23****	0.33****	0.19****	0.32****	0.26****	1.00****			
Limited mobility	<0.01	0.28****	0.17****	0.20****	0.33****	0.17****	0.19****	1.00****		
Numbness	0.03	0.26****	0.18****	0.23****	0.32****	0.23****	0.19****	0.42****	1.00****	
Pain	-0.07*	0.19****	0.01	0.14****	0.21****	0.20****	0.20****	0.46****	0.34****	1.00****

Bolded values indicate significance.

*p < 0.05;

***p < 0.001;

****p < 0.0001.

Three components or "clusters" were identified by the PCA at baseline. As shown in Table 4, the first component accounts for 3.4 units of total variance (equals to 10), the second component accounts for 1.6 units and the third accounts for 1.0 units of total variance. Therefore, the PCA extracted three components with eigenvalues greater than 1.0 and each component explained more than 10% of the variance. Cluster 1 was composed of anxiety, depression, exhaustion, and sleep interference. Cluster 2 included limited mobility, numbness, and pain. Cluster 3 consisted of constipation, digestion problems and headache. The first three components respectively accounted for 34%, 16%, and 10% of the total variance. Cumulatively, these components accounted for 60% of the total variance.

The three clusters showed good internal consistency with Cronbach's alpha values of 0.71, 0.67 and 0.64, respectively (see Table 5). The final communality estimates ranged from 0.40 (headache) to 0.74 (anxiety), indicating the variables were well accounted for by the three components.

The biplot between components 1 and 2, as well as the biplot between components 2 and 3, clearly indicate the three identified clusters (see Figure 1).

Table 4. Eigenvalues and proportions of variance for 10 components

Component	Eigenvalue	Proportion (%)	Cumulative (%)
1	**3.4**	**33.9**	**33.9**
2	**1.6**	**15.9**	**49.9**
3	**1.0**	**10.3**	**60.1**
4	0.8	7.9	68.0
5	0.7	6.6	74.6
6	0.6	6.2	80.9
7	0.6	5.8	86.6
8	0.5	5.0	91.6
9	0.5	4.9	96.5
10	0.3	3.5	100.0

Clusters identified in the principle component analysis (PCA) are bolded.

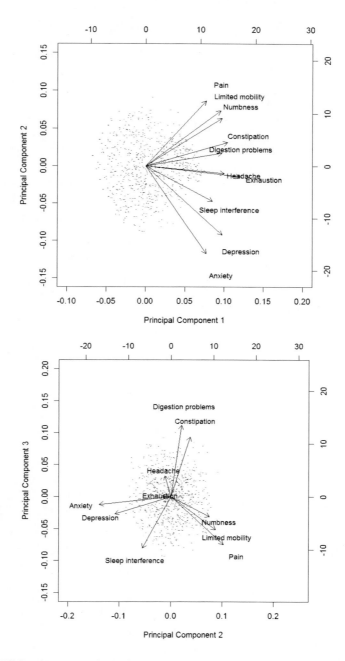

Figure 1. Biplots between principal components 1 and 2, 2 and 3.

Table 5. Factor loadings and final communality

Symptom	Component 1	Component 2	Component 3	Final communality
Anxiety	**0.83**	-0.17	0.15	0.74
Depression	**0.81**	0.03	0.18	0.68
Exhaustion	**0.48**	0.34	0.44	0.54
Sleep interference	**0.65**	0.32	-0.04	0.52
Limited mobility	0.08	**0.75**	0.20	0.61
Numbness	0.10	**0.66**	0.28	0.52
Pain	0.01	**0.80**	0.05	0.64
Constipation	0.06	0.21	**0.79**	0.67
Digestion problems	0.07	0.09	**0.82**	0.69
Headache	0.34	0.20	**0.49**	0.40
% of variance	34%	16%	10%	
Cronbach's alpha	0.71	0.67	0.64	

Bolded values indicate inclusion of symptoms in respective components.

DISCUSSION

There is little research investigating the demographic and symptom profiles of medical cannabis patients. A study conducted in California reported that the majority of patients using medical cannabis were male, Caucasian, between the ages 25-44 years, and employed (8). A similar demographic profile was also seen in the present study, with the majority of patients being male and Caucasian.

In the present study, the PCA produced three symptom clusters at baseline. The first cluster (anxiety, depression, exhaustion and sleep interference) has been commonly studied in cancer patients (9). In a sample of patients undergoing chemotherapy, Redeker et al. (10) reported a significant negative impact of insomnia, fatigue, anxiety and depression on quality of life (p<0.001) (10). Sleep interference in particular has been indicated as an exacerbating factor in symptom clusters, contributing to a further decrease in quality of life. Fatigue and sleep interference are issues not limited to cancer patients, as they have been frequently reported in patients with multiple sclerosis and a number of other chronic conditions (11-12).

There is partial overlap between prevalent conditions observed in the present study and those reported by Ware et al. (13) in their nationwide survey of medical cannabis users in the United Kingdom. The authors reported cannabis use in patients with chronic pain, multiple sclerosis, depression, arthritis, and neuropathy. Similarly, the most prevalent conditions reported in the present study sample included chronic pain and depression, along with sleep disorders, anxiety disorder, and post-traumatic stress disorder.

There is existing evidence of the efficacy of medical cannabis in treating these particular conditions. In another analysis of self-reported medical cannabis use and effectiveness, Bonn-Miller et al. reported its particular helpfulness in treating psychological symptoms and anxiety (14). A systematic review and meta-analysis of 18 trials conducted by Martin-Sanchez et al. suggested cannabis may be efficacious in managing chronic pain (15). A more recent review conducted by Jensen et al. reported strong evidence in support of cannabinoids for the treatment of cancer-related pain, particularly at mid-range doses (16). The authors remarked on the reduction in pain and improvement in sleep quality following cannabis treatment in this patient population. Recent discussion has also suggested the use of cannabis may be a safer and effective therapeutic alternative to conventional opioids for the treatment of chronic pain (17).

A more thorough understanding of symptom clustering in patients using medical cannabis may help healthcare providers more effectively manage symptomatology. With more research on the efficacy of different strains for the management of specific symptoms, clusters can be targeted and effectively managed with minimization of poly-pharmacy and potentially associated side-effects.

CONCLUSION

Medical cannabis patients often present with a variety of symptoms, such as pain, sleep interference, and anxiety. Symptoms reported by medical cannabis patients in a voluntary online survey were grouped into three distinct clusters. The understanding of symptom clusters in medical cannabis patients may allow more targeted treatment of concurrent symptoms with specific strains. Further research on the symptom profile of this patient population, and strain efficacy for different indications is required for more sensitive and effective management of symptoms.

ACKNOWLEDGMENT

We thank the generous support of Bratty Family Fund, Michael and Karyn Goldstein Cancer Research Fund, Joey and Mary Furfari Cancer Research Fund, Pulenzas Cancer Research Fund, Joseph and Silvana Melara Cancer Research Fund, and Ofelia Cancer Research Fund. This study was conducted in collaboration with MedReleaf.

REFERENCES

[1]   Chow E, Fan G, Hadi S, Filipczak L. Symptom clusters in cancer patients with bone metastases. Support Care Cancer 2007;15:1035-43.
[2]   Fan G, Filipczak L, Chow E. Symptom clusters in cancer patients: a review of the literature. Curr Oncol 2007;14(5):173-9.
[3]   Kimble LP, Dunbar SB, Weintraub WS, McGuire DB, Manzo SF, Strickland OL. Symptom clusters and health-related quality of life in patients with chronic stable angina. J Adv Nurs 2011;67(5):1000-11.
[4]   Yu DSF, Chan HYL, Leung DYP, Hui E, Sit JWH. Symptom clusters and quality of life among patients with advanced heart failure. J Geriatr Cardiol 2016;13(5):408-14.
[5]   Wong A, Lau AYL, Yang J, Wang Z, Liu WM, Lam BYK et al. Neuropsychiatric symptom clusters in stroke and tranisent ischemic attack by cognitive status and stroke subtype. PLoS One 2016;11(9):e0162846.
[6]   Grotenhermen F, Muller-Vahl K. The therapeutic potential of cannabis and cannabinoids. Dtsch Arztebl Int 2012;109(29-30):495-501.

[7]   Kruskal JB. Nonmetric multidimensional scaling by optimizing goodness of fit to a nonmetric hypothesis. Psychometrika 1964;29:1-27.

[8]   Nunberg HL, Kilmer B, Pacula RL, Burgdorf J. An analysis of appicants presenting to a medical marijuana specailty practic ein California. J Drug Policy Anal 2011;4(1):1-14.

[9]   Fiorentino L, Rissling M, Liu L, Ancoli-Israel S. The symptom cluster of sleep, fatigue, and depressive symptoms in breast cancer patients: severity of the problem and treatment options. Drug Discov Today Dis Models 2011;8(4):167-73.

[10]   Redeker NS, Lev EL, Ruggiero J. Insomnia, fatigue, anxiety, depression, and quality of life cancer patients undergoing chemotherapy. Scholarly Inquiry for Nursing Practice 2000;14(4):275-90.

[11]   Nociti V, Losavio FA, Gnoni V, Losurdo A, Testani E, Vollono C et al. Sleep and fatigue in multiple sclerosis: a questionnaire-based, cross-sectional, cohort study. J Neurol Sci 2017;372:387-92.

[12]   Swain MG. Fatigue in chronic disease. Clinical Science 2000;99(1):1-8.

[13]   Ware MA, Adams H, Guy GW. The medicinal use of cannabis in the UK: results of a nationwide survey. Int J Clin Pract 2005; 59(3):291-5.

[14]   Bonn-Miller MO, Boden MT, Bucossi MM, Babson KA. Self-reported cannabis use characteristics, patterns and helpfulness among medical cannabis users. Am J Drug Alcohol Abuse 2014;40(1):23-30.

[15]   Martin-Sanchez, Furukawa TA, Taylor J, Martin JLR. Systematic review and meta-analysis of cannabis treatment for chronic pain. Pain Med 2009;10(8):1353-68.

[16]   Jensen B, Chen J, Furnish T, Wallace M. Medical marijuana and chronic pain: a review of basic science and clinical evidence. Curr Pain Headache Rep 2015;19(50):1-9.

[17]   Carter GT, Javaher SP, Nguyen MH, Garret S, Carlini BH. Re-branding cannabis: the next generation of chronic pain medicine? Pain Manag 2015;5(1):13-21.

In: Medical Cannabis   ISBN: 978-1-53611-907-7
Editors: S. O'Hearn, A. Blake et al. © 2017 Nova Science Publishers, Inc.

Chapter 4

THE USE OF MEDICAL CANNABIS
IN CANCER PATIENTS

Pearl Zaki[1], BSc(C), Alexia Blake[2], MSc,
Amiti Wolt[2], BA, Stephanie Chan[1], BSc(C),
Liying Zhang[1], PhD, Bo Angela Wan[1], MPhil,
Henry Lam[1], MLS, Carlo DeAngelis[1], PharmD,
Marissa Slaven[3], MD, Erynn Shaw[3], MD,
Vithusha Ganesh[1], BSc(C), Leila Malek[1], BSc(Hons),
Edward Chow[1], MBBS and Shannon O'Hearn[2],*, MSc
[1]Odette Cancer Centre, Sunnybrook Health Sciences Centre,
University of Toronto, Toronto, Ontario, Canada
[2]MedReleaf, Markham, Ontario, Canada
[3]Juravinski Cancer Centre, Hamilton Health Sciences,
Hamilton, Ontario, Canada

Therapeutic applications of medical cannabis within the cancer population, particularly for pain, treatment-related nausea and vomiting,

* Correspondence: Ms Shannon O'Hearn MSc, MedReleaf Corp, Markham Industrial Park, Markham ON, Canada. E-mail: sohearn@medreleaf.com.

and loss of appetite, have been investigated by few studies. In this chapter we examine the efficacy of cannabis treatment for symptom relief among cancer patients receiving cannabis treatment from a single Canadian medical cannabis provider. Data was obtained from a voluntary online survey that consisted of questions related to demographic information, current medical conditions, presence and severity of symptoms, and quality of life (QOL). Follow-up (FU) surveys were completed at 4 and 10 months following initial use. 164 patients reported a current or previous diagnosis of cancer, of which the most common types of primary tumours were gastrointestinal (17.7%, n=29), breast (13.4%, n=22), leukemia and lymphoma (13.4%, n=22), gynaecologic (9.2%, n=15), prostate (7.3%, n=12), and lung (7.3%, n=12). While improvements were seen in commonly reported symptoms, including pain, depression, anxiety, exhaustion, and sleep problems, the observations were not statistically significant. Statistical significance was demonstrated in patients' ability to cope with pain at 4-month FU (p<0.0001). QOL was stable from baseline to 4-month FU, where most reported good QOL (66.7%). Of associated QOL factors, only experience with sleep was found to be improved with statistical significance (p = 0.02). Side effects of cannabis use included dry mouth, psychoactive effects, decreased concentration and memory, and sleepiness. Further studies are needed to determine the efficacy of medical cannabis in comparison to conventional first-line therapies for management of symptoms in cancer patients in both short- and long-term treatment.

INTRODUCTION

Cancer patients suffer from a range of disease- and treatment-related symptoms that negatively impact quality of life (QOL), the most common of which include pain, treatment-related nausea and vomiting, and loss of appetite. In particular, cancer-related pain can severely affect 70-90% of those with advanced cancers (1). The standard treatment for cancer pain is currently opioids; however, some patients continue to experience inadequate pain relief despite opioid therapy and the use of other common adjuvant analgesics (1-4). In the current literature, various studies have investigated clinical utility of cannabis as a potential treatment for a number of cancer-related symptoms including pain, nausea and vomiting, lack of appetite, and difficulty with sleep (2-4). However, confounding findings in the literature draw attention to the need for further investigation. To best guide clinical decision-making, it is important to determine potential benefits, adverse effects, drug interactions, and effective routes of administration and dosing of medical cannabis prior to implementation for therapeutic uses in the cancer setting.

Cannabinoids are the most well-known constituents of the *Cannabis sativa L* plant with over 60 unique compounds identified to date. Due to their potent biological activity, delta-9-tetrehydrocannabinol (THC) and cannabidiol (CBD) are the two most well-studied cannabinoids. While THC is known primarily for its psychoactive effects, it has also been shown to provide analgesic, anti-emetic, anti-inflammatory, muscle relaxant, and appetite stimulating properties (1, 2). In comparison, CBD provides anti-convulsive, muscle relaxant, anxiolytic, and anti-inflammatory properties (1, 2). Some studies have also suggested that CBD can counter-act the paranoia and anxiety sometimes induced by THC, possibly through modulatory effects (1, 2). This pharmacologic activity follows the activation of CB-1 and CB-2 receptors. These receptors are part of the endocannabinoid system, which has been shown to naturally influence and assist with the regulation of mood, sleep, memory, appetite, and emotions via activation by endogenous ligands (1-3). In this chapter we investigate the possible benefits and side effects of the use of medical cannabis for symptom management and relief among cancer patients.

OUR RESEARCH

Patients beginning cannabis treatment with a single Canadian medical cannabis provider completed a voluntary online survey at baseline, which is defined as the time of registration with the provider. Those who completed the survey at baseline were invited to complete a follow-up (FU) survey after four months. Similarly, those who completed the 4-month FU survey were prompted to complete a second FU survey at 10 months after baseline.

The survey was designed by the medical cannabis provider using scientific literature as well as guidance from health care professionals with experience using medical cannabis for patient care. The questions were adapted from the literature to accommodate the wide range of patients surveyed. Pain was measured using the numeric rating scale. Additionally, an adaptation of the Pain Self-Efficacy Questionnaire was incorporated to determine perceived ability to cope with pain. QOL assessment was based on validated and commonly used screening tools.

The survey consisted of over 100 questions presented in a dynamic format customized to individual responses, where responses determine the subsequent questions asked (e.g., if a patient is not experiencing pain, no further pain-related questions are asked). Patients were given the choice to skip any question. As such, each patient completing the survey answered a unique set of questions and each question received different numbers of responses.

Demographic information, including age, sex, ethnicity, and employment status was collected at baseline. Patients were asked to identify any present medical conditions, including duration and severity of the conditions. For reported conditions, patients were asked FU questions specific to the condition to better characterize each patient's medical history. Patients who reported a diagnosis of cancer were asked to specify cancer type and stage.

Patients were also asked to report on any present symptoms related to medical conditions and classify the severity of symptoms as mild, moderate, or severe. If patients indicated the presence of pain, they were asked to rate their pain on a scale of 1 to 10, where 1 represented dull pain and 10 represented severe pain. In the absence of pain, patients reported 'no pain' and no further questions were asked. Ability to cope with pain was measured on a categorical scale using the following options: 'very easy,' 'somewhat easy,' 'somewhat difficult,' and 'very difficult.' Patients were also asked to report other current medications, specifying the name and dose, as well as any use of cannabis (previous or current) prior to beginning treatment with the cannabis supplied by the medical cannabis provider.

Patients were asked to rate their QOL using one of the following options: "very good," "good," "fair," "bad," or "very bad," as well as to indicate their perceived ability to perform activities of daily living (ADLs) with the options "very capable," "somewhat capable," "somewhat incapable," "very incapable," or "unsure." Additional questions assessed patients' current experiences with sleep, appetite, concentration, bowel activity, and sexual function based on difficulty, using the options "severe difficulty," "moderate difficulty," "no difficulty," "good," and "very good." Experiences with mobility and ability to dress and shower independently were also examined based on difficulty, with possible options ranging from severe, moderate, minimal, to no difficulty. General mood was assessed using the options "very positive," "positive," "neutral," "negative," and "very negative."

Follow-up (FU) surveys were completed at 4 months and 10 months following the completion of the baseline survey. Patients were asked to report any changes in present medical conditions following cannabis use (from the options "significant deterioration," "moderate deterioration," "slight deterioration," "no change," "slight improvement," "moderate improvement," or "significant improvement") as well as the time taken to achieve the change, if any. Information regarding medical cannabis use from the cannabis provider, including strains used, frequency of consumption, and methods of consumption, was collected. If present, pain was measured on a scale of 1 to 10. Ability to cope with pain following use of medical cannabis was measured using the similarly to baseline, using the options: "very easy," "somewhat easy," "somewhat difficult," or "very difficult." Questions regarding QOL were also repeated from baseline. Additionally, patients were asked to report any side effects experienced as a result of cannabis use, including type of side effect, frequency, duration, and severity.

Baseline and FU surveys were completed between January 2015 and October 2016. Only patients reporting a diagnosis of cancer who completed the survey at baseline and FU at 4 or 10 months were included for analysis in this study.

Descriptive analysis was conducted using proportions for categorical variables. The Fisher test or Chi-squared test was used as appropriate to determine significant association between pain severity and ability responses from baseline to follow-up visits, between improvement status (improvement, no change, or deterioration), and the presence of most common medical conditions, symptoms, and QOL. Changes in pain scores between baseline and FU were compared using paired t-tests. Two-sided p-value <0.05 was considered statistically significant. All analyses were conducted using Statistical Analysis Software (SAS version 9.4, Cary, NC).

FINDINGS

Of the 2,573 patients who completed the survey at baseline, 164 patients reported a current or previous diagnosis of cancer. Among cancer patients, the majority were male (56.1%) and Caucasian (82.7%) with an average age of 54.9 years. The most commonly reported primary cancers included gastrointestinal (17.7%, n=29), breast (13.4%, n=22), leukemia and lymphoma (13.4%, n=22), gynaecologic (9.2%, n=15), prostate (7.3%, n=12), and lung (7.3%, n=12). Additionally, the most common comorbidities included arthritis (20.4%, n=29), depression (16.2%, n=23), anxiety (13.4%, n=12), post-traumatic stress disorder (PTSD) (9.2%, n=13), and sleep disorder (7.0%, n=10). Most patients reported previous cannabis use (56.3%, n=81) and current use of cannabis at baseline (73.8%, n=62). All demographic information is presented in Table 1.

Patients who reported experiencing pain ranked their pain on a scale of 1 to 10 at baseline and 4-month FU, where a score of 1-4 represented mild pain, 5-7 represented moderate pain, and 8-10 represented severe pain. At baseline, recurring pain was present in 75.0% (n=140) of 160 cancer patients who responded to the question. Of the patients who reported on their pain at both baseline and 4-month FU (n=24), the proportion of those experiencing severe pain was reduced from 45.8% (n=11) to 16.7% (n=4), however the differences were not statistically significant (p=0.06). Since very few patients answered this question at baseline and 10-month FU, the results from 10-month FU were not included.

Table 1. Patient demographics

Demographic	n (%)
Gender (Total n=164)	
Male	92 (56.1%)
Female	72 (43.9%)
Age (Total n=164) in years	
≤18	2 (1.2%)
19-29	4 (2.4%)
30-39	20 (12.2%)
40-49	22 (13.4%)
50-59	46 (28.0%)
60-69	45 (27.4%)
≥70	25 (15.2%)
Ethnicity (Total n=162)	
Caucasian	134 (82.7%)
Spanish/Hispanic/Latino	2 (1.2%)
Native Canadian	11 (6.8%)
Black/African American	1 (0.6%)
Asian	2 (1.2%)
Prefer not to answer	6 (3.7%)
Other	6 (3.7%)
Other conditions (Total n=142)	
Arthritis	29 (20.4%)
Depression	23 (16.2%)
Anxiety	19 (13.4%)
PTSD	13 (9.2%)
Sleep disorder	10 (7.0%)
Previous cannabis use (Total n=144)	
Yes	81 (56.3%)
No	55 (38.2%)
Prefer not to answer	8 (5.6%)
Current cannabis use (Total n=62)	
Yes	62 (73.8%)
No	22 (26.2%)

Table 1. (Continued)

Demographic	n (%)
Primary cancer (Total n=164)	
Breast	22 (13.4%)
Prostate	12 (7.3%)
Lung	12 (7.3%)
Gastrointestinal	29 (17.7%)
Gynecologic	15 (9.2%)
Skin	5 (3.1%)
Osteosarcoma	3 (1.8%)
Urothelial	5 (3.1%)
Brain	7 (4.3%)
Leukemia and lymphoma	22 (13.4%)
Hepatocellular	3 (1.8%)
Male reproductive cancers	2 (1.2%)
Thyroid	5 (3.1%)
Other	22 (13.4%)
Cancer stage (Total n=159)	
Remission	47 (29.6%)
0	5 (3.1%)
1	10 (6.3%)
2	13 (8.2%)
3	21 (13.2%)
4	48 (30.2%)
Unknown	15 (9.4%)

PTSD: Post-traumatic stress disorder.

Twelve patients reported on ability to cope with pain at both baseline and 4-month FU. Seven patients reported 'very difficult' at baseline versus 0 patients at 4-month FU. These findings demonstrated statistically significant improvement in ability to cope with pain from baseline to 4-month FU (n=12, $p<0.0001$). Table 2 illustrates changes in pain scores and the ability to deal with pain in patients who responded at baseline and FU.

Table 2. Changes in pain severity and the ability to cope with pain at baseline and 4-month FU

	Baseline n (%)	4-month FU n (%)	P-value*
Pain severity (Total n=24)			
Mild	6 (25.0%)	13 (54.2%)	0.06
Moderate	7 (29.2%)	7 (29.2%)	
Severe	11 (45.8%)	4 (16.7%)	
Ability to cope (Total n=12)			
Very easy	1 (8.3%)	5 (41.7%)	**< 0.0001**
Somewhat easy	2 (16.7%)	4 (33.3%)	
Somewhat difficult	2 (16.7%)	3 (25.0%)	
Very difficult	7 (58.3%)	0 (0.0%)	

*Bolded values represent statistical significance ($p < 0.05$).

Table 3. Improvement in medical conditions at 4-month FU

Medical condition	Improvement n (%)	No change n (%)	Deterioration n (%)	p-value
Arthritis (Total n = 9)	5 (55.6%)	3 (33.3%)	1 (11.1%)	0.9
Depression (Total n = 7)	5 (71.4%)	2 (28.6%)	0 (0.0%)	0.7
Anxiety (Total n = 3)	2 (66.7%)	1 (33.3%)	0 (0.0%)	0.8
PTSD (Total n = 5)	5 (100.0%)	0 (0.0%)	0 (0.0%)	0.07
Sleep disorder (Total n = 7)	4 (57.1%)	2 (28.6%)	1 (14.3%)	0.9

Table 3 presents improvements in medical conditions with responses grouped into improvement (significant, moderate, or slight), no change, and deterioration (significant, moderate, or slight). Improvement was reported by 5 of 5 patients for PTSD (100.0%), 5 of 7 patients (71.4%) for depression, 2 of 3 patients (66.7%) for anxiety, 4 of 7 patients (57.1%) for sleep disorder, and 5 of 9 patients (55.6%) for arthritis. However, the results did not demonstrate statistically significant change.

Improvements in symptoms

The most common symptoms reported by patients were anxiety, depression, exhaustion, sleep problems, and weakness, as illustrated in Table 4. Table 5 demonstrates changes in symptoms at 4-month FU with responses grouped into improvement (signification, moderate, or slight), no change, and deterioration (signification, moderate, or slight). Patients reported changes in symptoms at 4-month FU and also rated the extent of change. Of the patients who responded at both baseline and 4-month FU, anxiety improved in 83.3% (n=24), depression improved in 58.3% (n=16), exhaustion improved in 25.0% (n=15), sleep problems improved in 66.7% (n=16), and weakness improved in 41.7% (n=15). However, these findings were not statistically significant.

Table 4. Symptom severity at baseline

Symptom	Severity		
	Mild n (%)	Moderate n (%)	Severe n (%)
Anxiety (Total n=116)	36 (31.0%)	70 (60.3%)	10 (8.6%)
Depression (Total n=91)	43 (47.3%)	33 (36.3%)	15 (16.5%)
Exhaustion (Total n=97)	17 (17.5%)	51 (52.6%)	29 (29.9%)
Sleep problems (Total n=108)	22 (20.4%)	58 (53.7%)	28 (25.9%)
Weakness (Total n=86)	25 (29.1%)	40 (46.5%)	21 (24.4%)

Table 5. Improvements in symptoms at four months

Symptom	Improvement n (%)	No change n (%)	Deterioration n (%)	p-value
Anxiety (Total n=24)	20 (83.3%)	3 (12.5%)	1 (4.2%)	0.3
Depression (Total n=16)	14 (58.3%)	2 (8.3%)	0 (0.0%)	0.1
Exhaustion (Total n=15)	6 (25.0%)	5 (20.8%)	4 (16.7%)	0.05
Sleep problems (Total n=23)	16 (66.7%)	5 (20.8%)	2 (8.3%)	0.7
Weakness (Total n=15)	10 (41.7%)	3 (12.5%)	2 (8.3%)	0.9

Improvement in quality of life (QOL)

The survey measured overall QOL and associated QOL factors such as mobility, ability to dress and shower independently, ability to perform ADLs, and general mood; Table 6 illustrates responses from patients at both baseline and 4-month FU. From baseline to 4-month FU, QOL and associated QOL factors remained stable. Notably, however, there was an observed overall decline in general mood; of the 33 patients who responded at both baseline and 4-month FU, 19 (57.6%) reported having a 'positive' mood at baseline compared to only 7 (21.2%) at 4-month FU. Only changes in general mood were found to be significant (p=0.02).

Patients also described their experiences with appetite, sleep, concentration, bowel activity, and sexual function based on difficulty. Table 7 shows the responses of patients who responded to this question at baseline and 4-month FU. Slight improvement in experiences with these factors was demonstrated between baseline and 4-month FU; however, the findings were only statistically significant for experiences with sleep (p=0.02) and sexual function (p=0.01).

Side effects

Nine patients reported the occurrence of side effects experienced due to cannabis use at 4-month FU, the most common of which were dry mouth, psychoactive effects, decreased memory, decreased concentration, and sleepiness; findings are demonstrated in table 8. Specifically, 4 of 9 reported dry mouth (44.4%), psychoactive effects (44.4%), and decreased memory (44.4%), 3 reported sleepiness (33.3%), and 2 reported decreased concentration (22.2%).

Pearl Zaki, Alexia Blake, Amiti Wolt et al.

**Table 6. Quality of life (QOL) and associated factors at baseline
and follow-up**

Response	Time Point		p-value*
	Baseline **n (%)**	**4 months** **n (%)**	
Quality of life (Total n=33)			
Very good	3 (9.1%)	3 (9.1%)	0.9
Good	16 (48.5%)	16 (16.5%)	
Fair	11 (33.3%)	12 (36.4%)	
Bad	3 (9.1%)	1 (3.0%)	
Very bad	0 (0.0%)	1 (3.0%)	
Mobility (Total n=32)			
No difficulty	9 (28.1%)	11 (34.4%)	0.9
Minimal difficulty	14 (43.8%)	11 (34.4%)	
Moderate difficulty	7 (21.9%)	8 (25.0%)	
Severe difficulty	2 (6.3%)	2 (6.3%)	
Ability to dress/shower independently (Total n=33)			
No difficulty	22 (66.7%)	23 (69.7%)	0.2
Minimal difficulty	9 (27.3%)	4 (12.1%)	
Moderate difficulty	2 (6.1%)	5 (15.2%)	
Severe difficulty	0 (0.0%)	1 (3.0%)	
Ability to perform ADL (Total n=33)			
Very capable	15 (45.5%)	22 (66.7%)	0.4
Somewhat capable	10 (30.3%)	8 (24.2%)	
Somewhat incapable	4 (12.1%)	1 (3.0%)	
Very incapable	3 (9.1%)	1 (3.0%)	
Don't know	1 (3.0%)	1 (3.0%)	
General mood (Total n=33)			
Positive	19 (57.6%)	7 (21.2%)	**0.02**
Neutral	8 (24.2%)	15 (45.5%)	
Negative	5 (15.1%)	9 (27.3%)	
Very negative	1 (3.0%)	2 (6.1%)	

*Bolded values represent statistical significance ($p < 0.05$); ADL: Activities of daily
  living.

Table 7. Experience with quality of life factors

Response	Time Point		p-value*
	Baseline **n (%)**	**4 months** **n (%)**	
Appetite (Total n=24)			
Very good	7 (29.2%)	9 (37.5%)	0.7
Good	4 (16.7%)	6 (25.0%)	
No difficulty	3 (12.5%)	3 (12.5%)	
Moderate difficulty	10 (41.7%)	6 (25.0%)	
Severe difficulty	0 (0.0%)	0 (0.0%)	
Sleep (Total n=22)			
Very good	0 (0.0%)	2 (9.1%)	**0.02**
Good	2 (9.1%)	6 (27.3%)	
No difficulty	1 (4.6%)	4 (18.2%)	
Moderate difficulty	16 (72.7%)	10 (45.5%)	
Severe difficulty	3 (13.4%)	0 (0.0%)	
Concentration (Total n=24)			
Very good	4 (16.7%)	7 (29.2%)	0.1
Good	7 (29.2%)	5 (20.8%)	
No difficulty	1 (4.2%)	5 (20.8%)	
Moderate difficulty	12 (50.0%)	6 (25.0%)	
Severe difficulty	0 (0.0%)	1 (4.2%)	
Bowel activity (Total n=23)			
Very good	7 (30.4%)	4 (17.4%)	0.8
Good	7 (30.4%)	7 (30.4%)	
No difficulty	4 (17.4%)	5 (21.7%)	
Moderate difficulty	4 (17.4%)	5 (21.7%)	
Severe difficulty	1 (4.4%)	2 (8.7%)	
Sexual function (n=23)			
Very good	1 (4.4%)	2 (8.7%)	**0.01**
Good	3 (13.0%)	8 (34.8%)	
No difficulty	3 (13.0%)	4 (17.4%)	
Moderate difficulty	8 (34.8%)	9 (39.1%)	
Severe difficulty	8 (34.8%)	0 (0.0%)	

*Bolded values represent statistical significance ($p < 0.05$).

Table 8. Side effects at follow-up

Side effect	Time point	
	4 months (Total n=9) n (%)	10 months (Total n=3) n (%)
Dry mouth	4 (44.4%)	2 (66.7%)
Psychoactive effects	4 (44.4%)	1 (33.3%)
Decreased memory	4 (44.4%)	1 (33.3%)
Decreased concentration	2 (22.2%)	2 (66.7%)
Sleepiness	3 (33.3%)	1 (33.3%)

DISCUSSION

The present study reviewed the results of a voluntary online survey administered by a Canadian medical cannabis provider to cancer patients. The efficacy of medical cannabis to treat cancer-related symptoms has been explored by few studies which have predominantly focused on nausea, appetite, and pain. Cannabis has been previously evaluated for potential analgesic use in cancer-associated pain, which was the most commonly reported symptom among patients in the present study. A randomized control trial (RCT) conducted by Noyes et al. with 10 cancer patients of various diagnoses found that the analgesic effect of higher doses of THC (between 15 to 20 mg) was significantly superior to placebo, however with greater reports of sedation (5). The limitations of the study include a small sample size as well as the fact that the 10 patients in the study were also concurrently receiving their regular analgesics with either the THC or placebo, which may have confounded the findings of the study (5).

Portenoy et al. also conducted an RCT using 360 patients with advanced cancer and opioid-refractory pain to examine the efficacy of nabiximols, a new cannabinoid oromucosal spray containing a 1:1 THC and CBD combination (6). Low (1-4 sprays/day) and medium (6-10 sprays/day) doses of nabiximols demonstrated improved analgesia superior to placebo after 5 weeks, however higher (11-16 sprays/day) doses were not found to be more effective than lower doses (6). Another study by Johnson et al. assessed the effects of cannabis extract preparations containing THC and CBD in varying ratios in 177 advanced cancer patients with uncontrolled pain despite long-term use of opioids (1). The study consisted of 3 arms: THC:CBD extract (n=60), THC extract (n = 58), and placebo (n=59). Pain relief was greatest in the THC:CBD arm as double the number of patients reported a 30% reduction in pain compared to placebo. The THC arm and placebo arm were comparable. These studies suggest there is a potential role for THC and CBD combinations in the treatment of cancer-related opioid-refractory pain.

Loss of appetite is another common symptom among cancer patients that can impact QOL. In the present study, patients demonstrated slight improvement in experiences with appetite at 4-month FU; however, these results were not statistically significant, likely due to the small sample size. Few RCTs have investigated the effects of THC on appetite and weight loss; however, of those few, it has been found that oral THC can stimulate appetite and slow down chronic weight loss in advanced cancer patients (4, 7). Jatoi et al. also studied the effects of cannabis on appetite in 469 adults with advanced cancer who had experienced weight loss of ≥2.3 kg or caloric intake of <20 calories/kg/day (7). 159 patients were placed on oral megestrol, a steroid progestin, 152 patients were placed on oral THC, and 158 patients received a combination of the two. The study reported that megestrol alone stimulated appetite in 75% of patients and induced weight in gain in 11%; whereas, oral THC alone stimulated appetite in 49% patients and induced weight gain in 3%. The combined treatment did not show any additional benefits. The differences observed were statistically significant. However, the study was criticized for using low doses of THC, which may have impacted the outcomes. These findings highlight the importance of investigating which doses are most effective for treating different symptoms, such as loss of appetite, prior to implementation of cannabis as a first-line or alternative treatment option for symptoms such as loss of appetite.

Cannabis is also known for its antiemetic properties. In the present study, while nausea and vomiting were not among the five most commonly reported symptoms, 35.1% (n=27) of the 77 patients who reported nausea and 67.5% (n=25) of the 40 patients who reported vomiting rated these symptoms as severe. The efficacy of cannabis on chemotherapy-induced nausea and vomiting (CINV) has been investigated in some studies. A meta-analysis by Amar lists 15 RCTs involving 600 total patients that compared nabilone, a synthetic cannabinoid-based medication, to placebo or other common anti-emetic drugs as a first-line agent (3). The findings demonstrated that nabilone is more effective compared to prochlorperazine, domperidone, and alizapride and preferred for continuous use by patients (3).

The present study demonstrated improvements in pain, QOL, and a variety of symptoms over the course of cannabis treatment, but only found statistically significant improvements in ability to cope with pain and experiences with sleep. Statistically significant changes were also found in general mood, where the change represented decline in mood; within the context of cancer, this finding is likely suggestive of disease-related changes among patients. The study at present has several limitations. The compliance rate was very low, especially at FU intervals. The small sample sizes of those responding at both baseline and FU limited the power of the statistical analysis. It is also possible that there was a higher incidence of responses with patients experiencing more positive outcomes, resulting in a positive skew in the data. The survey also did not include validated questionnaires specific to cancer. FU surveys were not consistently completed at exactly 4 and 10 months from baseline by all patients. Invites were sent at each time point, and responses were received between 4 and 10 months, and any time after 10 months for the 4 and 10 month FU surveys, respectively. Moreover, at baseline, approximately 74% of patients reported current cannabis use; therefore, any changes observed at FU are likely to be more representative of the changes in cannabis treatment. Self-reported information on concurrent medications, including type and dose, was incomplete and therefore not available for analyses, limiting the ability to identify any further confounding factors. The study was also unable to account for any adverse events over the course of treatment. Additionally, while those invited to complete FU surveys had active prescriptions at baseline, it is not known whether they had continued to fill prescriptions to remain on cannabis treatment.

CONCLUSION

The present study demonstrated improvements in pain, QOL, and a variety of symptoms, but only found statistically significant improvements in ability to cope with pain and experiences with sleep. Further studies are required to investigate the potential uses and side effects of medical cannabis in comparison to current first-line therapies. Studies should also consider factors for both short- and long-term treatment to best guide future clinical practices.

ACKNOWLEDGMENTS

We thank the generous support of Bratty Family Fund, Michael and Karyn Goldstein Cancer Research Fund, Joey and Mary Furfari Cancer Research Fund, Pulenzas Cancer Research Fund, Joseph and Silvana Melara Cancer Research Fund, and Ofelia Cancer Research Fund. This study was conducted in collaboration with MedReleaf.

REFERENCES

[1]   Johnson JR, Burnell-Nugent M, Lossignol D, Ganae-Motan ED, Potts R, Fallon MT. Multicenter, double-blind, randomized, placebo-controlled, parallel-group study of the efficacy, safety, and tolerability of THC:CBD extract and THC extract in patients with intractable cancer-related pain. J Pain Symptom Manage 2010;39(2):167–79.

[2]   Birdsall SM, Birdsall TC, Tims LA. The use of medical marijuana in cancer. Curr Oncol Rep 2016;18(7):40.

[3]   Amar BM. Cannabinoids in medicine: A review of their therapeutic potential. J Ethnopharmacol 2006;105(1-2):1–25.

[4]   Wilkie G, Sakr B, Rizack T. Medical marijuana use in oncology. JAMA Oncol 2016;2(5):670-5.

[5]   Noyes R, Brunk SF, Baram DA, Canter A. Analgesic effect of delta-9-tetrahydrocannabinol. J Clin Pharmacol 1975;15(2–3):139–43.

[6]   Portenoy RK, Ganae-Motan ED, Allende S, Yanagihara R, Shaiova L, Weinstein S, et al. Nabiximols for opioid-treated cancer patients with poorly-controlled chronic pain: A randomized, placebo-controlled, graded-dose trial. J Pain 2012;13(5):438–49.

[7]   Jatoi A, Windschitl HE, Loprinzi CL, Sloan JA, Dakhil SR, Mailliard JA, et al. Dronabinol versus megestrol acetate versus combination therapy for cancer-associated anorexia: a North Central Cancer Treatment Group study. J Clin Oncol 2002;20(2):567–73.

In: Medical Cannabis   ISBN: 978-1-53611-907-7
Editors: S. O'Hearn, A. Blake et al. © 2017 Nova Science Publishers, Inc.

Chapter 5

THE USE OF MEDICAL CANNABIS IN COMMON MEDICAL CONDITIONS EXCLUDING CANCER

*Pearl Zaki[1], BSc(C), Vithusha Ganesh[1], BSc(C),
Shannon O'Hearn[2], MSc, Amiti Wolt[2], BA,
Stephanie Chan[1], BSc(C), Liying Zhang[1], PhD,
Henry Lam[1], MLS, Bo Angela Wan[1], MPhil,
Marissa Slaven[3], MD, Erynn Shaw[3], MD,
Carlo DeAngelis[1], PharmD, Leila Malek[1], BSc(Hons),
Edward Chow[1], MBBS and Alexia Blake[2,*], MSc*
[1]Odette Cancer Centre, Sunnybrook Health Sciences Centre,
University of Toronto, Toronto, Ontario, Canada
[2]MedReleaf, Markham, Ontario, Canada
[3]Juravinski Cancer Centre, Hamilton Health Sciences,
Hamilton, Ontario, Canada

---

* Correspondence: Ms Alexia Blake, MSc, MedReleaf Corp, Markham Industrial Park, Markham ON, Canada. E-mail: ablake@medreleaf.com.

The potential clinical utility of medical cannabis in the management of a wide variety of symptoms and conditions is gaining increasing attention. In this chapter we investigate possible benefits and side effects associated with the use of cannabis in patients diagnosed with non-cancer-related conditions. All patients received cannabis from a single Canadian medical cannabis provider. 2,588 patients completed a voluntary online survey prior to the initiation of cannabis use, defined as baseline. Follow-up (FU) surveys were completed at 4 and 10 months after baseline. The survey collected information pertaining to patient demographics, medical conditions, presence and severity of symptoms, and quality of life (QOL). The most commonly reported medical conditions other than cancer were anxiety disorder (32.9%, n=713), depression (32.6%, n=706), sleep disorders (26.7%, n=579), post-traumatic stress disorder (PTSD) (22.6%, n=489), and arthritis (22.5%, n=488). At 4-month FU, a majority of patients demonstrated improvement in all conditions: arthritis (70.0%, n=98), anxiety (77.5%, n=162), depression (71.6%, n=211), sleep disorders (79.2%, n=154) and PTSD (76.9%, n=160), with significant improvements seen in anxiety (p=0.0006), PTSD (p=0.006), and sleep disorders (p=0.0006). Reductions in symptoms and symptom severity, as well as improvement in QOL were also demonstrated at 4-month FU and remained stable from 4-month to 10-month FU. Pain severity was significantly reduced from baseline to 10-month FU (p<0.0001). To achieve optimal patient outcomes, future studies should investigate the efficacy of medical cannabis including effects of different cannabis varieties, doses, and methods of consumption when used for various medical conditions.

INTRODUCTION

Medical cannabis has been investigated for the potential to provide a variety of therapeutic benefits. Current literature and anecdotal accounts suggest that cannabis is most commonly used to reduce nausea and vomiting, stimulate appetite, assist with sleep, and relieve pain (1, 2). However, thorough clinical investigation is required to fully understand the intricacies of using medical cannabis in a clinical setting, with a focus on safety and efficacy. This information will be valuable to both patients and physicians, and help guide clinical decision-making.

The pharmacological properties of cannabis make it well-suited for potential uses in the treatment of various conditions and symptoms.

Cannabis contains over 60 cannabinoids, with tetrahydrocannabinol (THC) and cannabidiol (CBD) being the two most well-known examples. THC is the major psychoactive component of cannabis and is known to possess analgesic, anti-emetic, appetite stimulating, and muscle relaxant properties (1,2). Cannabidiol (CBD) is another well-studied cannabinoid that has demonstrated anti-convulsant, anxiolytic, and anti-inflammatory effects (1,2). The present study examined possible benefits and adverse effects associated with the use of medical cannabis for therapeutic applications in common medical conditions, with the exception of cancer, through a voluntary online survey.

OUR STUDY

Patients receiving cannabis treatment completed a voluntary online survey designed by a Canadian medical cannabis supplier. Participating patients completed the survey at baseline (i.e., the time of registration with the cannabis provider). Those who completed the survey at baseline were invited to complete a follow-up (FU) survey at four months from baseline and similarly, those who completed the survey at four months were prompted to complete a second FU survey at 10 months from baseline.

The survey consisted of over 100 questions presented in a dynamic format customized to individual responses, where responses determined the subsequent questions asked (e.g., if a patient was not experiencing pain, no further pain-related questions were asked). Patients were also given the choice to skip questions. As such, each patient completing the survey answered a unique set of questions and each question received different numbers of responses.

The survey was developed using scientific literature and in collaboration with health care professionals with experience prescribing medical cannabis for patient care. The questions were modified from the literature to accommodate a wide range of patients. Pain was measured using the numeric rating scale. An adaptation of the Pain Self-Efficacy Questionnaire was included in the survey to determine perceived ability to cope with pain. Assessments of quality of life (QOL) were adapted from validated and commonly used screening tools.

Demographic information, including age, sex, ethnicity, and employment status was collected at baseline. Patients were asked to identify any present medical conditions, including duration and severity of the conditions, as well as to report on the presence and severity of any symptoms related to medical conditions. If patients indicated the presence of recurring pain, they were subsequently asked to rate their pain on a scale of 1 to 10, where 1 represented dull pain and 10 represented severe pain. Ability to cope with pain was measured using the options: "very easy," "somewhat easy," "somewhat difficult," and "very difficult." Patients were also asked to report any other current medications as well as previous experience with cannabis, including the frequency of use and method of consumption, if any.

Patients were asked to rate their overall QOL using the options "very good," "good," "fair," "bad," and "very bad" and indicate their perceived ability to perform activities of daily living (ADLs) from the options "very capable," "somewhat capable," "somewhat incapable," "very incapable," or "unsure." Mobility and ability to dress/shower independently were measured based on difficulty ranging from no, minimal, moderate, to severe difficulty. General mood was assessed using the options "very positive," "positive," "neutral," "negative," or "very negative." Additional questions assessed patients' current experiences with sleep, appetite, concentration, bowel activity, and sexual function, where patients were able to select from the options "severe difficulty," "moderate difficulty," "no difficulty," "good," or "very good" to represent their experience.

Follow-up

FU surveys were completed at 4 months and 10 months from baseline. To assess the response to medical cannabis, patients were asked to rate the effect of cannabis on present medical conditions, by categorizing the status of their conditions as one of the following: "significant deterioration," "moderate deterioration," "slight deterioration," "no change," "slight improvement," "moderate improvement," and "significant improvement," as well as the time taken to achieve the change, if any. Questions regarding medical cannabis use including frequency of and methods of consumption were repeated from baseline. Patients were also asked to report which cannabis strains they had used. If present, pain was measured on a scale of 1 to 10 and ability to cope was categorized using the same options as presented at baseline. Questions regarding QOL were repeated from baseline. Additionally, patients were asked to report any side effects experienced as a result of cannabis use, including type of side effect, frequency, duration, and severity.

Baseline and FU surveys were completed between January 2015 and December 2016. Patients reporting non-cancer conditions who completed surveys at minimum at baseline and 4 month FU were included.

Descriptive analysis was conducted using proportions for categorical variables. The Fisher test or Chi-squared test was used as appropriate to determine significant association between pain severity and ability to cope with pain responses from baseline to FU, and between improvement status (improvement, no change, or deterioration) and the presence of the most common medical conditions, QOL, and symptoms. Changes in pain scores between baseline and FU were compared using paired two-tailed t-tests. A p-value <0.05 was considered statistically significant. All analyses were conducted using Statistical Analysis Software (SAS version 9.4, Cary, NC).

OUR FINDINGS

2,588 of the 2,752 patients who completed the survey at baseline reported medical conditions other than cancer. The majority of patients were Caucasian (79.2%) and male (69.2%) with an average age of 42.7 years. The most commonly reported medical conditions included anxiety disorder (32.9%, n=713), depression (32.6%, n=706), sleep disorders (26.7%, n=579), post-traumatic stress disorder (PTSD) (22.6%, n=489), and arthritis (22.5%, n=488). 1772 patients (76.8%) reported previous cannabis use, while 366 patients (15.9%) reported no previous cannabis use and 170 patients (7.37%) preferred not to answer. Current cannabis use at baseline was reported by 86.2% of patients (n=1492). Table 1 illustrates all patient demographics.

Table 1. Patient demographics

Demographic	n (%)
Gender (Total n=2753)	
Male	1790 (69.2%)
Female	798 (30.8%)
Age in years (Total n=2753)	
≤18	22 (1.7%)
19-29	403 (15.6%)
30-39	713 (27.6%)
40-49	563 (21.6%)
50-59	571 (22.1%)
60-69	237 (9.2%)
≥70	57 (2.2%)
Ethnicity (Total n=2601)	
Caucasian	2060 (79.2%)
Spanish/Hispanic/Latino	20 (0.8%)
Native Canadian	123 (4.7%)
Black/African American	41 (1.6%)
Asian	45 (1.7%)
Other	312 (12.0%)
Other conditions (Total n=2165)	
Anxiety	713 (32.9%)
Depression	706 (32.6%)
Sleep disorder	579 (26.7%)
PTSD	489 (22.6%)
Arthritis	488 (22.5%)
Previous cannabis use (Total n=2821)	
Yes	1772 (76.8%)
No	366 (15.9%)
Prefer not to answer	170 (7.4%)
Current cannabis use (Total n=1730)	
Yes	1492 (86.2%)
No	238 (13.8%)

PTSD: Post-traumatic stress disorder.

Patients reported pain severity on a scale of 1 to 10, from which scores were categorized into mild (1-4), moderate (5-7), and severe (8-10). 30.2% of patients (n=633) reported pain at baseline with the majority rating their pain as severe (n=68, 61.3%). Notably, severe pain was reduced from 61.3% (n=68) of patients at baseline to 10.8% (n=12) at 4-month FU and 6.31% (n=7) at 10-month FU. Changes in pain severity were found to be statistically significant (p<0.0001) at all-time points.

Sixty-seven patients reported their ability to cope with pain at all-time points (baseline, 4-month FU, and 10-month FU). From baseline, the proportion of those who reported ability to cope as 'very easy' increased from 0% of patients to 20.8% (n=14) at 4-month FU and 25.4% (n=17) at 10-month FU. Similarly, those who reported ability to cope as 'very difficult' decreased from 64.2% of patients (n=43) at baseline to 1.49% (n=1) at 4-month FU and remained stable at 10-month FU. Changes in ability to cope with pain were statistically significant (p<0.0001) between baseline and 4-month and 10-month FUs. Table 2 demonstrates changes in pain severity and ability to cope with pain at all-time points.

Responses for changes in medical conditions were more broadly categorized into improvement (comprising slight, moderate, and significant), no change, and deterioration (comprising slight, moderate, and medium). These results are presented in Table 3. Improvements were observed in all major conditions including sleep disorder (79.2%, n=122), anxiety (77.5%, n=162), PTSD (76.9%, n=122), depression (71.6%, n=151), and arthritis (70.0%, n=98). Statistical significance was demonstrated for anxiety (p=0.0006), PTSD (p=0.006), and sleep disorder (n=0.0006).

Patients reported on frequently experienced symptoms and their severity at baseline, the most common of which were pain, anxiety, depression, exhaustion, and sleep problems. At baseline, patients predominantly reported severe pain (50.3%, n=950), moderate anxiety (49.0%, n=923), moderate depression (45.8%, n=706), moderate exhaustion (47.4%, n=832), and moderate sleep problems (45.9%, n=832). Symptom severity at baseline is illustrated in Table 4.

Table 2. Changes in pain severity and the ability to cope with pain at baseline and FU

	Baseline, n (%)	4-month FU, n (%)	10-month FU, n (%)	p-value*
Pain severity (Total n=111)				
Mild	9 (8.1%)	53 (47.8%)	71 (64.0%)	**< 0.0001**
Moderate	34 (30.6%)	46 (41.4%)	33 (29.7%)	
Severe	68 (61.3%)	12 (10.8%)	7 (6.3%)	
Ability to cope (Total n=67)				
Very easy	0 (0%)	14 (20.8%)	17 (25.4%)	**< 0.0001**
Somewhat easy	2 (3.0%)	40 (59.7%)	38 (56.7%)	
Somewhat difficult	22 (32.8%)	12 (17.9%)	11 (16.4%)	
Very difficult	43 (64.2%)	1 (1.5%)	1 (1.5%)	

*Bolded values represent statistical significance (p < 0.05).

Table 3. Improvement in medical conditions at 4-month FU

Medical condition	Improvement, n (%)	No change, n (%)	Deterioration, n (%)	p-value*
Arthritis (Total n=140)	98 (70.0%)	23 (16.4%)	19 (13.6%)	0.6
Depression (Total n=211)	151 (71.6%)	34 (16.1%)	26 (12.3%)	0.2
Anxiety (Total n=209)	162 (77.5%)	17 (8.1%)	30 (14.4%)	**0.0006**
PTSD (Total n=160)	123 (76.9%)	17 (10.6%)	20 (12.5%)	**0.007**
Sleep disorder (Total n=154)	122 (79.2%)	17 (11.0%)	15 (9.7%)	**0.0006**

*Bolded values represent statistical significance (p < 0.05).
PTSD: Post-traumatic stress disorder.

Table 4. Symptom severity at baseline

Symptom	Severity		
	Mild, n (%)	Moderate, n (%)	Severe, n (%)
Pain (Total n=1887)	172 (9.1%)	765 (40.5%)	950 (50.3%)
Anxiety (Total n=1882)	495 (26.3%)	923 (49.0%)	464 (26.7%)
Depression (Total n=1541)	493 (32.0%)	706 (45.8%)	342 (22.2%)
Exhaustion (Total n=1289)	354 (27.4%)	611 (47.4%)	324 (25.1%)
Sleep problems (Total n=1814)	360 (19.8%)	832 (45.9%)	622 (34.3%)
Weakness (Total n=870)	383 (44.0%)	384 (44.1%)	103 (11.8%)

Table 5. Improvements in symptoms at FU

Symptom	Deterioration, n (%)	No change, n (%)	Improvement, n (%)	Resolved, n (%)	p-value*
4-month FU					
Pain (Total n=435)	33 (7.6%)	49 (11.3%)	346 (79.5%)	7 (1.6%)	**0.002**
Anxiety (Total n=432)	38 (8.8%)	63 (14.5%)	323 (74.8%)	8 (1.9%)	0.06
Depression (Total n=364)	40 (11.0%)	65 (17.9%)	250 (68.7%)	9 (2.5%)	0.9
Exhaustion (Total n=305)	21 (6.9%)	95 (31.1%)	181 (59.3%)	8 (2.6%)	0.1
Sleep Problems (Total n=423)	33 (7.8%)	60 (14.2%)	315 (74.5%)	15 (3.6%)	**0.01**
Weakness (Total n=183)	22 (12.0%)	60 (32.8%)	89 (48.6%)	12 (6.6%)	0.06
10-month FU					
Pain (Total n=113)	6 (5.3%)	17 (15.0%)	84 (74.3%)	6 (5.3%)	0.5
Anxiety (Total n=103)	10 (9.7%)	12 (11.7%)	77 (74.8%)	4 (3.9%)	0.4
Depression (Total n=85)	5 (5.9%)	7 (8.2%)	66 (77.6%)	7 (8.2%)	0.6

Table 5. (Continued)

Symptom	Deterioration, n (%)	No change, n (%)	Improvement, n (%)	Resolved, n (%)	p-value*
Exhaustion (Total n=70)	5 (7.1%)	19 (27.1%)	44 (62.9%)	2 (2.9%)	0.7
Sleep Problems (Total n=105)	7 (6.7%)	7 (6.7%)	83 (79.0%)	8 (7.6%)	0.8
Weakness (Total n=47)	3 (6.4%)	18 (38.3%)	24 (51.1%)	2 (4.6%)	0.7

*Bolded values represent statistical significance (p<0.05).

Changes in experiences of symptoms and symptom severity were measured at 4-month and 10-month FU using the following options: deterioration, no change, improvement, or resolved, as demonstrated in Table 5. Improvement was reported in 79.5% of patients (n=346) for pain, 74.8% (n=323) for anxiety, 68.7% (n=250) for depression, 59.3% (n=181) for exhaustion, 74.5% (n=315) for sleep problems, and 48.6% (n=89) for weakness. Between 1-7% of patients reported complete resolution of symptoms at 4-month FU, including anxiety (1.9%, n=8), depression (2.5%, n=9), exhaustion (2.6%, n=8), sleep problems (3.6%), and weakness (6.6%, n=12). Changes in pain (p=0.002) and sleeping problems (p=0.01) were found to be statistically significant. At 10-month FU, improvement in symptoms ranged from approximately 51% to 79%, however, none were found to be statistically significant.

Improvement in quality of life (QOL)

Patients reported changes in QOL and associated QOL indicators, which included mobility, ability to dress/shower independently, ability to perform activities of daily living (ADLs), and general mood from baseline to 4-month and 10-month FU, as shown in Table 6. Reports of "very good" QOL were increased from 4.8% of patients (n=6) at baseline to 14.5% (n=18) at 4-month FU and 13.7% (n=17) at 10-month FU. From baseline to

4-month FU, a greater proportion of patients reported "good" QOL (increased from 22.6% to 33.9%) and a smaller proportion reported "fair" (decreased from 45.2% to 41.1%), "bad" (decreased from 22.6% to 8.9%), or "very bad" (decreased from 4.8% to 1.6%) QOL; however there was little difference in QOL between 4-month and 10-month FU. Changes reported in QOL from baseline to 4-month and 10-month FU were statistically significant (p=0.001). Of the associated QOL indicators, only changes in general mood were found to be statistically significant. Compared to 5.0% of patients (n=6) at baseline, "very positive" general mood was reported by 12.4% (n=15) at 4-month FU and 14.9% (n=18) at 10-month FU.

Table 6. Quality of life and associated factors at baseline and FU

Response	Time point			p-value*
	Baseline **n (%)**	**4-month** **FU** **n (%)**	**10-month** **FU** **n (%)**	
Quality of life (Total n=124)				
Very good	6 (4.8%)	18 (14.5%)	17 (13.7%)	**0.001**
Good	28 (22.6%)	42 (33.9%)	44 (35.5%)	
Fair	56 (45.2%)	51 (41.1%)	46 (37.1%)	
Bad	28 (22.6%)	11 (8.9%)	16 (12.9%)	
Very bad	6 (4.8%)	2 (1.6%)	1 (0.8%)	
Mobility (Total n=119)				
No difficulty	34 (28.6%)	39 (32.8%)	45 (37.8%)	0.1
Minimal difficulty	32 (26.9%)	41 (34.5%)	25 (21.0%)	
Moderate difficulty	43 (36.1%)	33 (27.7%)	43 (36.1%)	
Severe difficulty	10 (8.4%)	6 (5.0%)	6 (5.0%)	
Ability to dress/shower independently (Total n=121)				
No difficulty	65 (53.7%)	71 (58.7%)	69 (57.0%)	0.9
Minimal difficulty	37 (30.6%)	36 (29.8%)	35 (28.9%)	
Moderate difficulty	18 (14.9%)	13 (10.7%)	17 (14.0%)	
Severe difficulty	1 (0.8%)	1 (0.8%)	0 (0.0%)	

Table 6. (Continued)

Ability to perform ADL (Total n=124)				
Very capable	50 (40.3%)	47 (37.9%)	47 (37.9%)	0.4
Somewhat capable	39 (31.5%)	52 (41.9%)	49 (39.5%)	
Somewhat incapable	25 (20.2%)	20 (16.1%)	16 (12.9%)	
Very incapable	9 (7.26%)	5 (4.0%)	11 (8.9%)	
Don't know	1 (0.8%)	0 (0.0%)	1 (0.8%)	
General mood (Total n=121)				
Very positive	6 (5.0%)	15 (12.4%)	18 (14.9%)	**< 0.001**
Positive	43 (35.5%)	55 (45.5%)	53 (43.8%)	
Neutral	41 (33.9%)	47 (38.8%)	34 (28.1%)	
Negative	27 (22.3%)	2 (1.7%)	15 (12.4%)	
Very negative	4 (3.3%)	2 (1.7%)	1 (0.8%)	

*Bolded values represent statistical significance ($p < 0.05$).
ADL: Activities of daily living.

Patients were also asked about changes in experiences with other QOL indicators including appetite, sleep, concentration, bowel activity, and sexual function, the findings of which are illustrated in Table 7. Improved experiences were observed in each of the QOL indicators. From baseline to 4-month FU, reports of 'very good' experiences increased from 20% to 26.4% of patients for appetite, 2.8% to 19.3% for sleep, 8.2% to 19.1% for concentration, 10.8% to 27.0% for bowel activity, and 16.3% to 26.0% for sexual function. 'Very good' experiences were notably reduced for concentration at 10-month FU (10.9%), however 'good' experiences improved from 20.9% of patients to 35.5% of patients from 4-month to 10-month FU in this outcome. Otherwise, most experiences with QOL factors remained stable between 4-month and 10-month FU. Only findings for experiences with sleep and concentration were found to be statistically significant ($p < 0.001$ and p=0.002 respectively).

Side effects

The most commonly reported side effects included dry mouth, psychoactive effects, decreased memory, decreased concentration, and sleepiness. 23 patients reported side effects at both 4-month and 10-month FU, as illustrated in Table 8. At 4-month FU, 16 (69.6%) reported dry mouth, 15 (65.2%) reported psychoactive effects, 12 (35.3%) reported decreased memory and concentration, and 11 (32.4%) reported sleepiness. At 10-month FU, reports of side effects were decreased for dry mouth (63.9%), psychoactive effects (50.0%), and decreased concentration (33.3%), but increased for decreased memory (36.1%) and sleepiness (44.4%). Patients also reported on severity of side effects at FU; the results at 4-month FU are displayed in Table 9. A majority of patients reported mild dry mouth (45.9%, n=39), mild psychoactive effects (45.5%, n=30,), mild decreased memory (56.7%, n=17), mild decreased concentration (60.0%, n=21), and moderate sleepiness (46.8%, n=22).

Table 7. Experience with quality of life factors at baseline and FU

Response	Time point			p-value*
	Baseline, n (%)	4-month FU, n (%)	10-month FU, n (%)	4-month FU n (%)
Appetite (Total n=110)				
Very good	22 (20.0%)	29 (26.4%)	31 (28.2%)	0.4
Good	32 (29.1%)	40 (36.4%)	36 (32.7%)	
No difficulty	21 (19.1%)	17 (15.5%)	22 (20.0%)	
Moderate difficulty	27 (24.5%)	19 (17.3%)	18 (16.4%)	
Severe difficulty	8 (7.3%)	5 (4.5%)	3 (2.7%)	
Sleep (Total n=109)				
Very good	3 (2.8%)	21 (19.3%)	14 (12.8%)	**< 0.001**
Good	3 (2.8%)	21 (19.3%)	32 (29.4%)	
No difficulty	3 (2.8%)	10 (9.2%)	8 (7.3%)	
Moderate difficulty	59 (54.1%)	43 (39.4%)	40 (36.7%)	
Severe difficulty	41 (37.6%)	14 (12.8%)	15 (13.8%)	

Table 7. (Continued)

Response	Time point			p-value*
	Baseline, n (%)	4-month FU, n (%)	10-month FU, n (%)	4-month FU n (%)
Concentration (Total n=110)				
Very good	9 (8.2%)	21 (19.1%)	12 (10.9%)	**0.002**
Good	22 (20.0%)	23 (20.9%)	39 (35.5%)	
No difficulty	17 (15.5%)	21 (19.1%)	17 (15.5%)	
Moderate difficulty	43 (39.1%)	38 (34.5%)	37 (33.6%)	
Severe difficulty	19 (17.3%)	7 (6.4%)	5 (4.5%)	
Bowel activity (Total n=23)				
Very good	22 (10.8%)	30 (27.0%)	24 (21.6%)	0.6
Good	31 (27.9%)	23 (20.7%)	30 (27.0%)	
No difficulty	26 (23.4%)	22 (19.8%)	25 (22.5%)	
Moderate difficulty	20 (18.0%)	29 (26.1%)	22 (19.8%)	
Severe difficulty	12 (19.8%)	7 (6.3%)	10 (9.0%)	
Sexual function (Total n=23)				
Very good	17 (16.3%)	27 (26.0%)	32 (30.8%)	0.1
Good	18 (17.3%)	24 (23.1%)	22 (21.2%)	
No difficulty	20 (19.2%)	22 (21.2%)	21 (20.2%)	
Moderate difficulty	29 (27.9%)	18 (17.3%)	18 (17.3%)	
Severe difficulty	20 (19.2%)	13 (12.5%)	11 (10.6%)	

*Bolded values represent statistical significance (p < 0.05).

Table 8. Side effects at 4-month and 10-month FU

Side effect	Time point	
	4-month FU (Total n=34), n (%)	10-month FU (Total n=36), n (%)
Dry mouth	24 (70.6%)	23 (63.9%)
Psychoactive effects	21 (61.8%)	18 (50.0%)
Decreased memory	12 (35.3%)	13 (36.1%)
Decreased concentration	12 (35.3%)	12 (33.3%)
Sleepiness	11 (32.4%)	16 (44.4%)

Table 9. Severity of side effects at 4-month FU

Side effect	Severity		
	Mild, n (%)	Moderate, n (%)	Severe, n (%)
Dry mouth (Total n=85)	39 (45.9%)	35 (41.2%)	11 (12.9%)
Psychoactive effects (Total n=66)	30 (45.5%)	29 (43.9%)	7 (10.6%)
Decreased memory (Total n=30)	17 (56.7%)	10 (33.3%)	3 (10.0%)
Decreased concentration (Total n=35)	21 (60.0%)	11 (31.4%)	3 (8.6%)
Sleepiness (Total n=47)	20 (42.3%)	22 (46.8%)	5 (10.6%)

DISCUSSION

The present study investigated the results of a voluntary online survey administered by a Canadian medical cannabis supplier, with the focus on the responses to cannabis use in patients with medical conditions excluding cancer. The goal of the study was to assess the efficacy of cannabis treatment for symptom management and relief in various medical conditions, of which the most common were anxiety, depression, sleep disorder, PTSD, and arthritis.

From the survey data collected, there was a statistically significant ($p<0.0001$) reduction in pain severity between baseline and 4 and 10-month FU. Similarly, patients reported an increase in their ability to cope with pain following cannabis use from baseline to 4 and 10-month FU ($p<0.0001$).

These findings are consistent with results of other studies found in the literature which examined the analgesic properties of cannabis. A thorough literature review conducted by Amar (1) identified nine controlled studies which have examined pain in patients with a variety of medical conditions excluding cancer (1). One of the identified studies was a randomized control trial (RCT) by Notcutt et al. (3) that examined the analgesic effects of THC and CBD in 34 patients with chronic pain (3). Patients were randomized to receive one of three varieties of cannabis-based extracts: THC, CBD, or 1:1 THC:CBD administered by a sublingual spray over a

12-week period. Two patients dropped out of the study; one was unable to cope with study requirements and the other was unable to tolerate the treatment. In the remaining 32 patients, extracts containing THC (THC alone and THC:CBD combination) demonstrated effective pain relief as well as improvements in sleep quality, while CBD alone was ineffective. Some minor side effects were observed, including dry mouth, drowsiness, euphoria/dysphoria, and dizziness.

Similar findings were reported by Berman et al. (4) in their RCT involving 48 patients with central neuropathic pain treated with either THC or THC:CBD sublingual spray for three periods of two weeks (4). Three patients withdrew prior to study completion, of which two experienced adverse effects of THC. The results of the 45 patients completing the study demonstrated a statistically significant decrease in pain and improvement in sleep quality with both the THC alone and the THC:CBD combination, with only mild to moderate side effects.

However, another RCT by Buggy et al. (5) examined the analgesic effect of oral THC in 40 women undergoing hysterectomies with post-operative pain and found no significant differences between treatment and placebo groups in mean summed pain intensity difference (SPID, primary outcome) 6 hours after intake (5). No significant adverse outcomes were observed with the dosage used in this study, thus future studies may consider the use of higher doses, while being cognizant that previous studies have indicated a higher incidence of adverse events with higher doses (1,5).

Notcutt et al. (3) and Berman et al. (4) demonstrated significant improvements in pain and sleep with mild to moderate side effects in patients suffering from chronic pain while Buggy et al. (5) did not find significant improvements among patients with post-operative or acute pain. This may suggest differences exist in the treatment of chronic and acute pain. In the present study, significant changes were found in the presence and severity of recurrent or chronic pain, however acute pain was not considered. Patients of this study also reported similar side effects to those observed by Noctcutt et al. (3) and Berman et al. (4), including dry mouth and psychoactive effects or euphoria/dysphoria. Further investigations should explore appropriate dosing, combinations of cannabinoids, and methods of consumption to assess the efficacy of cannabis as an analgesic for both chronic and acute pain.

Medical cannabis has also been indicated for appetite stimulation, particularly cancer- or AIDS-related anorexia-cachexia; however, present evidence is limited and further research is required to understand its potential role in the treatment of these conditions (1). Struwe et al. (6) studied the efficacy of cannabis for appetite stimulation in 12 men with symptomatic HIV and weight loss of >2.3 kg using 5 mg oral THC (6). Of the 12 patients, 2 experienced sedation and mood disorders and withdrew prior to completion. Out of the remaining 10 patients, THC was found to stimulate appetite but there was no statistically significant difference in weight variations between patients receiving THC or placebo. A larger study by Beal et al. (7) examined the use of oral THC in 139 patients with AIDS and weight loss of >2.3 kg and found a statistically significant stimulation of appetite and stabilization of weight in those using THC compared to those using the placebo (7). Only minor side effects were reported, including euphoria, dizziness, confusion, and drowsiness. In the present study, those with HIV/AIDS accounted for <1% (n=7) of all patients surveyed. While overall experiences with appetite for all patients (excluding cancer patients) demonstrated improvement from baseline to 10-month FU (20.0% reported 'very good' at baseline, 28.2% at 10-month FU), the changes were not statistically significant (p=0.4). This may have been due to the characteristics of the study population, many of which did not report loss or trouble with appetite. Only 7.3% (n=8) of surveyed patients reported severe difficulty with appetite at baseline. Further studies should investigate the efficacy of cannabis for appetite stimulation in particular study samples where appetite stimulation is an appropriate indication, for example cancer or HIV patients.

Cannabis has also demonstrated anti-spastic properties, which present potential therapeutic uses in the treatment of multiple sclerosis (MS) (1). Approximately 2% of the patients surveyed in the present study reported having MS. Zajicek et al. (8) studied the effects of oral THC on spasticity in 630 MS patients and found a small treatment effect on muscle spasticity as well as improvements in mobility, pain, sleep quality, and general condition (8). Wade et al. conducted a study in 160 MS patients using a 1:1 combination of THC:CBD administered via sublingual spray (9). They reported statistically significant reductions in spasticity with the THC:CBD combination compared to placebo, as well as significant improvements in sleep quality, but insignificant improvement in mobility.

Some anecdotal reports have also suggested that cannabis may function as an anti-convulsant, particularly in epilepsy and generalized tonic-clonic seizures (1). In this study, epilepsy was also observed in approximately 2% of patients surveyed. Cunha et al. (10) examined the efficacy of CBD in treating seizures in 15 patients with generalized epilepsy inadequately controlled by conventional medications (10). Of the eight patients randomized to receive CBD, 50% (n=4) remained convulsion-free over the duration of the study and 38% (n=3) demonstrated improvement. Drowsiness was reported by 50% of the patients on CBD. Overall, the evidence to support anti-spastic and anti-convulsant properties of cannabis remains low. Further investigation is required before cannabis may be implemented as effective treatment for conditions such as MS and epilepsy.

CBD is also known to produce anxiolytic effects, and therefore may be used in the treatment of anxiety disorders, insomnia, and epilepsy. Both sleep problems and anxiety were amongst the most commonly reported symptoms in this study. Carlini and Cunha (11) assessed the effects of 3 doses of CBD (40, 80, and 160 mg) in 15 insomniac patients and found a significant increase in the duration of sleep in those receiving 160 mg CBD (11). Findings in the present study also demonstrated significant improvement in experiences with sleep from baseline to 10-month FU ($p < 0.0001$). However, dose and variants of cannabis taken were not specified.

Another study by Fabre and McLendon (12) investigated the effects of nabilone, a synthetic cannabinoid mimicking THC, in 20 patients diagnosed with anxiety (12). Nabilone was found to be significantly more effective than placebo in relieving anxiety ($p < 0.0001$). While this study demonstrated improvements in anxiety at 4-month and 10-month FU

(74.8% improved at both 4-month FU and 10-month FU), the changes were not statistically significant (p=0.07 at 4-month FU, p=0.4 at 10-month FU).

The results of the present study indicate that cannabis may be used in the treatment of pain, anxiety, sleep disorders, as well as a number of other symptoms in patients suffering from a variety of medical conditions, excluding cancer. These findings are in general agreement with those reported in the literature. However, there are significant limitations in the present study that should be considered. Since the survey was completed on a voluntary basis, the compliance rate was very low. As such, despite having an initially large sample size at baseline, the results returned low numbers of responses for many of the parameters, especially at later FU intervals. The smaller sample sizes may have limited the power of the statistical analysis. It is also possible that there was a higher incidence of responses from patients experiencing more positive outcomes, resulting in a positive skew. Also, the time at which FU surveys were completed was not consistent between subjects, since patients may have completed FU surveys at any time after receiving a survey invitation. Moreover, at baseline, approximately 86% of patients reported current cannabis use; therefore, any changes observed at FU are possibly due to a change in cannabis treatment. Furthermore, since the data on concurrent medications, including type and dose, was self-reported, much of the information was incomplete and therefore not available for analysis. The study was also unable to account for any adverse events that occurred over the course of cannabis use. Finally, it is not known if those who were invited to complete FU surveys had continued to fill prescriptions from baseline to 10-month FU, although patients had active prescriptions at the time of invite.

CONCLUSION

Further clinical investigation is required to determine the utility of medical cannabis and support its use as an alternative or first-line treatment for a variety of common conditions and symptoms. Future studies should focus on the effects of different cannabis varieties, dosing, and methods of consumption as they pertain to different medical conditions in order to optimize patient outcomes.

ACKNOWLEDGMENTS

We thank the generous support of Bratty Family Fund, Michael and Karyn Goldstein Cancer Research Fund, Joey and Mary Furfari Cancer Research Fund, Pulenzas Cancer Research Fund, Joseph and Silvana Melara Cancer Research Fund, and Ofelia Cancer Research Fund. This study was conducted in collaboration with MedReleaf.

REFERENCES

[1]   Ben Amar M. Cannabinoids in medicine: A review of their therapeutic potential. J Ethnopharmacol 2006;105(1):1–25.

[2]   Zhornitsky S, Potvin S. Cannabidiol in Humans—The Quest for Therapeutic Targets. Pharmaceuticals 2012;5(12):529–52.

[3]   Notcutt W, Price M, Miller R, Newport S, Phillips C, Simmons S, et al. Initial experiences with medicinal extracts of cannabis for chronic pain: results from 34 "N of 1" studies. Anaesthesia 2004;59(5):440–52.

[4]   Berman JS, Symonds C, Birch R. Efficacy of two cannabis based medicinal extracts for relief of central neuropathic pain from brachial plexus avulsion: results of a randomised controlled trial. Pain 2004;112(3):299–306.

[5]   Buggy DJ, Toogood L, Maric S, Sharpe P, Lambert DG, Rowbotham DJ. Lack of analgesic efficacy of oral delta-9-tetrahydrocannabinol in postoperative pain. Pain 2003;106(1–2):169–72.

[6]   Struwe M, Kaempfer SH, Geiger CJ, Pavia AT, Plasse TF, Shepard K V, et al. Effect of dronabinol on nutritional status in HIV infection. Ann Pharmacother 1993;27(7–8):827–31.

[7]   Beal JE, Olson R, Laubenstein L, Morales JO, Bellman P, Yangco B, et al. Dronabinol as a treatment for anorexia associated with weight loss in patients with AIDS. J Pain Symptom Manage 1995;10(2):89–97.

[8]   Zajicek JP, Sanders HP, Wright DE, Vickery PJ, Ingram WM, Reilly SM, et al. Cannabinoids in multiple sclerosis (CAMS) study: safety and efficacy data for 12 months follow up. J Neurol Neurosurg Psychiatry 2005;76(12):1664–9.

[9]   Wade DT, Makela P, Robson P, House H, Bateman C. Do cannabis-based medicinal extracts have general or specific effects on symptoms in multiple sclerosis? A double-blind, randomized, placebo-controlled study on 160 patients. Mult Scler 2004;10(4):434–41.

[10]   Cunha JM, Carlini EA, Pereira AE, Ramos OL, Pimentel C, Gagliardi R, et al. Chronic administration of cannabidiol to healthy volunteers and epileptic patients. Pharmacology 1980;21(3):175–85.

[11]   Carlini EA, Cunha JM. Hypnotic and antiepileptic effects of cannabidiol. J Clin Pharmacol 1981;21(8–9 Suppl):417S–427S.

[12]   Fabre LF, McLendon D. The efficacy and safety of nabilone (a synthetic cannabinoid) in the treatment of anxiety. J Clin Pharmacol 1981;21(8–9 Suppl):377S–382S.

In: Medical Cannabis   ISBN: 978-1-53611-907-7
Editors: S. O'Hearn, A. Blake et al. © 2017 Nova Science Publishers, Inc.

Chapter 6

EFFICACY OF DIFFERENT VARIETIES
OF MEDICAL CANNABIS
IN RELIEVING SYMPTOMS

Bo Angela Wan[1], MPhil, Patrick Diaz[1], PhD(C),
Alexia Blake[2], MSc, Stephanie Chan[1], BSc(C),
Amiti Wolt[2], BA, Pearl Zaki[1], BSc(C),
Liying Zhang[1], PhD, Marissa Slaven[3], MD,
Erynn Shaw[3], MD, Carlo DeAngelis[1], PharmD,
Henry Lam[1], MLS, Vithusha Ganesh[1], BSc(C),
Leila Malek[1], BSc(Hons), Edward Chow[1], MBBS
and Shannon O'Hearn[2,*], MSc
[1]Odette Cancer Centre, Sunnybrook Health Sciences Centre,
University of Toronto, Toronto, Ontario, Canada
[2]MedReleaf, Markham, Ontario, Canada
[3]Juravinski Cancer Centre, Hamilton Health Sciences,
Hamilton, Ontario, Canada

---

[*] Correspondence: Ms. Shannon O'Hearn MSc, Project Manager, Clinical Research, MedReleaf, Markham Industrial Park, Markham, Ontario, Canada. E-mail: sohearn@medreleaf.com.

Traditionally, cultivars of *Cannabis sativa* L. have been divided into sub-species based on their morphological properties, metabolic profile, and geographical origin. Interbreeding subspecies renders hybrids characterised by varying *sativa* and *indica* profiles, and unique cannabinoid ratios. As cannabinoid compounds like tetrahydrocannabinol (THC) and cannabidiol (CBD) are thought to be primarily responsible for the physiological effects of cannabis, unique strain profiles may provide different therapeutic benefits suitable for managing different symptoms and conditions. This chapter aims to assess the efficacy of different cannabis varieties in patients using medical cannabis from one Canadian licensed provider. Information pertaining to current medical conditions, symptoms, and quality of life were collected through a voluntary online survey administered to patients after registration, and at 4 and 10 month follow-up intervals. 837 patients provided information about their experience with medical cannabis at 4-month follow-up. Patients reported that the variety *Midnight*^{MR} (*sativa*-leaning, 8-11% THC, 11-14% CBD) was most efficacious for reducing pain (27.4%), and that *Luminarium*^{MR} (very *sativa*-dominant, 25-28% THC, 0% CBD) was effective for managing both anxiety disorder (30.4%) and depression (35.5%). Patients most commonly attributed improvements in sleep (29.0%), appetite (24.8%), and bowel function (24.6%) to *Midnight*^{MR}, improvements in concentration (22.0%) to *Cognitiva*^{MR} (*sativa*-leaning, 15-18% THC, 0% CBD), and improvements in sexual function (26.5%) to *Luminarium*^{MR}. The efficacy of different cannabis varieties in managing various symptoms should be further investigated in a controlled clinical setting, to enable patients and physicians to make informed decisions on which varieties are best suited to achieve optimal symptom management.

INTRODUCTION

Cannabis contains over 421 different chemical compounds of several molecular classes, including flavonoids, terpenes, steroids, and cannabinoids. Of these compounds, cannabinoids are perhaps the most well studied group, in particular tetrahydrocannabinol (THC) and cannabidiol (CBD) (1). Both THC and CBD bind to endogenous cannabinoid receptors of the mammalian endocannabinoid system, resulting in a variety of downstream effects related to the modulation of mood, memory, appetite, pain, and inflammation (2). Thus, medical cannabis is used in the management of a variety of conditions and symptoms related to these modulatory effects, including pain, nausea and vomiting, depression, anxiety, and insomnia (3–5).

The physiological effects of cannabis are a product of the composition and concentration of active constituents found in each variety, as well as their complex pharmacological interactions and metabolism in the human body. In addition, the pharmacokinetics of cannabinoids also varies depending on the route of administration (4).

The endocannabinoid system contains two types of receptors known as CB-1 and CB-2. THC has an affinity for both receptor types, with a slight preference for CB-1 (2). CB-1 is found on the presynaptic membranes of neurons in the central and peripheral nervous system, as well as in peripheral tissues, such as the heart and spleen (6, 7). The activation of CB-1 receptors in the nervous system plays a role in cognition and pain signalling (2). CB-2 receptors are found mainly on cells of the immune system, and are the predominant cannabinoid receptors expressed by leukocytes. The activation of CB-2 receptors leads to a downregulation of the inflammatory response, which contributes to analgesic effects (6).

Because of the ability of THC to bind to both of these receptors and activate these different pathways, it is administered in the clinical setting for its analgesic, anti-emetic, anti-spastic, and psychotropic effects. Early clinical research suggests it may be efficacious in the management of symptoms such as chronic and neuropathic pain, and spasticity (8).

The molecular mechanism of CBD is less well understood, but it is thought to be polypharmacological. CBD is a weak antagonist of CB-1 receptors, and an agonist of the serotonergic 5-HT$_{1A}$ receptor, which is found in central and peripheral nervous systems and controls varying physiological and psychological pathways, including regulation of mood, appetite, and sleep (9). Some evidence exists that suggests CBD may have some effect on the metabolism of THC or on THC's interaction with the body's endocannabinoid system (10). The anti-inflammatory, anti-spastic, and anxiolytic effects of CBD lead to its use in the management of pain, insomnia, and epilepsy in the clinical setting (7, 11).

In addition to cannabinoids, terpenes are another important class of compounds thought to be associated with the physiological effects of the plant. 120 unique terpenes have been isolated in the cannabis plant (1). Terpenes produce their own range of pharmacological activities, and it is possible that they are equally, if not more important, than cannabinoids in terms of therapeutic effects. Clinical and anecdotal evidence suggest that the delivery of whole-plant products is more effective than isolated cannabinoids for symptom management. This is believed to be a consequence of synergistic interactions between cannabinoids, terpenes, and other plant constituents, often described as the "Entourage Effect" (12).

While cannabis speciation has been a topic of debate, the current scientific consensus is that it is a single species known as *Cannabis sativa* L. with three commonly recognized sub-species, *indica, sativa,* and *ruderalis* (13). Interbreeding of these subspecies has resulted in the creation of over 700 hybrid varieties that span the morphological and pharmacological characteristics of both *sativa* and *indica* plants (14). Different cannabis hybrids express differing cannabinoid ratios and terpene profiles. Moreover, identical strains grown in different environments may also produce different cannabinoid and terpene profiles. The varying physiological effects induced by *indica* and *sativa* strains leads to different clinical uses of cannabis varieties. For example, *indica* dominant varieties are traditionally associated with more sedative or relaxing effects, while *sativa* dominant varieties are thought to produce more stimulating or energizing effects (14).

Although numerous medical cannabis varieties are available, only anecdotal or self-reported evidence exists to suggest which strains are best indicated for the management of particular symptoms or conditions. Based on existing knowledge, doctors may recommend specific parameters on cannabinoid content or method of administration depending on a patient's condition or experience with the medication. Patients may also use a trial-and-error method to find a variety that works optimally for their specific condition or symptoms, and adjust strain and dosage depending on how and when it is administered (14). This selection process can be complicated by the fact that differences in every individual's biochemistry can play a role in their experience with the medication, as well as the fact that there is still a limited understanding of the role and interactions between terpenes and cannabinoids in vivo. Therefore, intensive investigation is required to better understand the clinical utility of different cannabis strains as a function of their unique chemical profiles.

The aim of the chapter was to assess patient reported efficacies of different cannabis varieties in managing their conditions and symptoms based on information provided through a voluntary online survey. These results will allow physicians to better recommend different strains of medical cannabis for future patients to more effectively and efficiently address their medical needs.

OUR STUDY

An online survey was designed by a Canadian medical cannabis provider in consultation with physicians and nurses experienced in prescribing medical cannabis, and with reference to relevant scientific literature. Existing validated questionnaires that assessed pain and quality of life were adapted to assess specific attributes of the target patient population. Questions assessing patients' pain levels were measured on a scale of 0-10 (with 0 being no pain and 10 being worst possible pain), and patients' ability to cope with their pain was assessed based on an adaption of the Pain Self-Efficacy Questionnaire (15). Quality of life (QOL) questions were based on two commonly used and validated methods of QOL assessment (16, 17). The survey was dynamic, and patients were given questions based on relevance as determined by their answers to earlier questions (e.g., patients were not asked about their pain experience if they did not indicate pain as a symptom or condition). Since the survey was customized to best assess each patient's unique characteristics, not all questions were mandatory and not all patients answered every question.

Patients of one licensed medical cannabis producer were invited to complete an intake survey at the time of registration, which is considered "baseline." The survey collected demographic information and information pertaining to current medical conditions and symptoms. Condition and symptom severity was reported as mild, moderate, or severe. Patients were asked additional detailed questions relevant to the symptoms or conditions they selected. QOL was assessed by asking patients to report on their experiences with items such as sleep, appetite, concentration, bowel activity, and sexual function, by selecting from the options "severe difficulty," "moderate difficulty," "no difficulty," "good," and "very good."

Patients were invited to complete a follow-up survey 4 and 10 months following completion of the initial intake survey. Patients were asked to report any changes they had experienced to their symptoms, conditions, or QOL. They were also asked about their experience with medical cannabis, and if they had experienced any changes in their symptoms or conditions, which of the cannabis varieties they perceived the changes could be attributed to. Cannabis varieties were categorized based on their approximate *sativa* and *indica* character. *Sativa*-leaning strains consist of 50-60% *sativa* character, *sativa*-dominant strains consist of 61-70% *sativa* character, and very *sativa*-dominant strains consist of >70% *sativa* character. *Indica* strains are similarly characterised.

Patients who completed surveys between January 2015 and January 2017 were included in this analysis. Baseline survey data was filtered to include only patients who indicated which strains they took at the 4-month follow-up for analysis.

FINDINGS

In total, 837 patients reported which cannabis varieties they consumed at 4-month follow-up. The demographic and lifestyle characteristics of these patients at baseline are presented in Table 1. The majority of patients were male (68.8%), Caucasian (83.4%), and reported that they have prior experience with cannabis at the time of survey completion (78.9%). The average age of patients was 44.9 years old, with an age range from one year to 80 years old. Most patients belonged in the age bracket of 50-59 (28.7%). The most common medical conditions reported in this patient cohort at baseline included depression (34.5%), anxiety disorder (34.3%), post-traumatic stress disorder (PTSD, 25.9%), and sleep disorder (25.7%). Pain was reported by 33.0% of patients at baseline. The most common symptoms at baseline included anxiety (40.7%), sleep problems (38.4%), depression (29.9%), insomnia (29.3%), and headache (20.4%).

Table 1. Baseline demographics of patients who indicated cannabis varieties associated with symptom improvement

Demographic	n (%)
Gender (Total n=837)	
Male	575 (68.8%)
Female	259 (30.9%)
Other	3 (0.4%)
Ethnicity (Total n=836)	
Caucasian	697 (83.4%)
Spanish/Hispanic/Latino	4 (0.5%)
Native Canadian	40 (4.8%)
Black/African American	8 (1.0%)
Asian	10 (1.2%)
Pacific Islander	1 (0.1%)
Prefer not to answer	31 (3.7%)
Other	45 (5.4%)
Age in years (Total n=833)	
0 - 19	22 (2.6%)
19 - 29	66 (7.9%)
30 - 39	209 (25.1%)
40 - 49	179 (21.5%)
50 - 59	239 (28.7%)
60 - 69	96 (11.5%)
≥70	22 (2.6%)
Average (min, max)	44.9 (1, 80)
Other conditions (Total n=837)	
Depression	289 (34.5%)
Anxiety disorder	287 (34.3%)
PTSD	217 (25.9%)
Sleep disorder	215 (25.7%)
Previous experience with cannabis (Total n=835)	
Yes	659 (78.9%)
No	118 (14.1%)
Prefer not to answer	58 (6.9%)

PTSD: Post-traumatic stress disorder.

651 patients reported on which cannabis varieties they felt contributed most to any improvements in overall health. These are presented in Table 2, along with information pertaining to each variety's composition, THC and CBD content, as well as price. The variety *Midnight^MR* (*sativa*-leaning, 8-11% THC, 11-14% CBD, $12.50/g) was the most popular strain overall, with 18.7% of all patients perceiving it to be the most beneficial cannabis strain contributing to improvements in overall health. This was followed by *Avidekel^MR* (*indica*-leaning, 0.1-0.8% THC, 15-18% CBD, $12.50/g) preferred by 13.7% of patients, and *Sedamen^MR* (*indica*-dominant, 21-24% THC, 0% CBD, $12.50/g) preferred by 9.4% of patients.

Table 2. Properties of 15 most popular cannabis strains perceived to be most beneficial overall

Strain	Patients found most beneficial, n (%)	Composition	% THC	% CBD	$/gram
Midnight^MR	122 (18.7%)	*sativa*-leaning	8 - 11%	11 - 14%	12.5
Avidekel^MR	89 (13.7%)	*indica*-leaning	0.1 - 0.8%	15 - 18%	12.5
Sedamen^MR	61 (9.4%)	*indica*-dominant	21 - 24%	0	12.5
Luminarium^MR	57 (8.8%)	*sativa*-dominant	25 - 28%	0	12.5
Cognitiva^MR	51 (7.8%)	*sativa*-leaning	15 - 18%	0	5
Remissio^MR	29 (4.5%)	*indica*-dominant	24 - 27%	0	12.5
Alaska^MR	26 (4.0%)	*sativa*-dominant	20 - 23%	0	15
Erez^MR	24 (3.7%)	*indica*-dominant	20 - 23%	0	7.5
Eran Almog^MR	20 (3.1%)	very *indica*-dominant	25 - 28%	0	15
Contenti^MR	16 (2.5%)	*indica*-leaning	15 - 18%	0	5
Cerebri^MR	14 (2.2%)	very *indica*-dominant	25 - 28%	0	12.5
Voluptas^MR	14 (2.2%)	very *sativa*-dominant	20 - 23%	0	12.5
Elevare^MR	13 (2.0%)	very *sativa*-dominant	24 - 27%	0	12.5
Stellio^MR	11 (1.7%)	*indica*-dominant	23 - 26%	0	12.5
Or^MR	10 (1.5%)	*indica*-dominant	20 - 23%	0	15

Improvements in conditions, symptoms, and QOL items

Table 3 lists the top five conditions reported by patients, and the three cannabis varieties to which improvements in conditions at 4-month follow up were attributed. These conditions include anxiety, depression, sleep disorder, arthritis, and post-traumatic stress disorder. Improvement was most commonly reported by patients experiencing anxiety as a condition at intake. Out of 69 patients, 35.5% attributed their anxiety reduction to the variety *Luminarium*^{MR} (very *sativa*-dominant, 25-28% THC, 0% CBD, $12.50/g). This was followed by *Midnight*^{MR} (27.5%) and *Avidekel*^{MR} (21.7%).

Table 3. Top three cannabis strains associated with condition improvement

Condition (Total n)	1st	2nd	3rd
	Luminarium^{MR}	*Midnight*^{MR}	*Avidekel*^{MR}
Anxiety disorder (69)	n=21 (30.4%)	n=19 (27.5%)	n=15 (21.7%)
	Luminarium^{MR}	*Avidekel*^{MR}	*Alaska*^{MR}
Depression (62)	n=22 (35.5%)	n=18 (29%)	n=16 (25.8%)
	Eran Almog^{MR}	*Sedamen*^{MR}	*Midnight*^{MR}
Sleep disorder (53)	n=17 (32.1%)	n=17 (32.1%)	n=11 (20.8%)
	Midnight^{MR}	*Avidekel*^{MR}	*Sedamen*^{MR}
Arthritis (46)	n=18 (39.1%)	n=15 (32.6%)	n=13 (28.3%)
	Stellio^{MR}	*Luminarium* ^{MR}	*Sedamen*^{MR}
PTSD (41)	n=15 (36.6%)	n=13 (31.7%)	n=12 (29.3%)

PTSD: Post-traumatic stress disorder.

Six of the most common symptoms for which patients reported improvements after 4 months of medical cannabis use include anxiety (as a symptom rather than condition), sleep problems, depression, insomnia, headaches, and exhaustion (Table 4). 27.3% of 341 patients attributed improvements in their symptom of anxiety to *Sedamen*^{MR}. This was followed by *Luminarium*^{MR} (25.2%), and *Cognitiva*^{MR} (22.0%). 27.7% out of 321 patients attributed improvements in sleep problems to *Luminarium*^{MR}, followed by *Midnight*^{MR} (24.6%), and *Avidekel*^{MR} (20.2%).

Table 4. Top three cannabis strains associated with symptom improvement

Symptom (Total n)	1st	2nd	3rd
Anxiety (341)	*Sedamen*[MR]	*Luminarium*[MR]	*Cognitiva*[MR]
	n=93 (27.3%)	n=86 (25.2%)	n=75 (22.0%)
Sleep problems (321)	*Luminarium*[MR]	*Midnight*[MR]	*Avidekel*[MR]
	n=89 (27.7%)	n=79 (24.6%)	n=65 (20.2%)
Depression (250)	*Luminarium*[MR]	*Avidekel*[MR]	*Alaska*[MR]
	n=80 (32%)	n=63 (25.2%)	n=50 (20%)
Insomnia (245)	*Eran Almog*[MR]	*Sedamen*[MR]	*Midnight*[MR]
	n=68 (27.8%)	n=61 (24.9%)	n=45 (18.4%)
Headache (171)	*Midnight*[MR]	*Avidekel*[MR]	*Sedamen*[MR]
	n=53 (31%)	n=40 (23.4%)	n=39 (22.8%)
Exhaustion (164)	*Stellio*[MR]	*Luminarium*[MR]	*Sedamen*[MR]
	n=43 (26.2%)	n=38 (23.2%)	n=29 (17.7%)

Table 5. Top three strains associated with QOL improvement

Symptom (Total n)	1st	2nd	3rd
Sleep (224)	*Midnight*[MR]	*Sedamen*[MR]	*Avidekel*[MR]
	n=65 (29.0%)	n=51 (22.8%)	n=37 (16.5%)
Appetite (302)	*Midnight*[MR]	*Cognitiva*[MR]	*Sedamen*[MR]
	n=75 (24.8%)	n=73 (24.2%)	n=69 (22.8%)
Concentration (191)	*Cognitiva*[MR]	*Midnight*[MR]	*Avidekel*[MR]
	n=42 (22.0%)	n=39 (20.4%)	n=37 (19.4%)
Bowel function (175)	*Midnight*[MR]	*Sedamen*[MR]	*Avidekel*[MR]
	n=43 (24.6%)	n=37 (21.1%)	n=36 (20.6%)
Sexual function (170)	*Luminarium*[MR]	*Sedamen*[MR]	*Cognitiva*[MR]
	n=45 (26.5%)	n=44 (25.9%)	n=36 (21.2%)

QOL: quality of life.

At the 4-month follow-up, patients were asked about which cannabis varieties they felt were responsible for changes, if any, in five quality of life measures, including sleep, appetite, concentration, bowel activity, and sexual function (see Table 5). 224 and 175 patients attributed improvements in sleep and bowel function to three specific strains: *Midnight*^{MR} (29.0% and 24.6%, respectively), *Sedamen*^{MR} (22.8% and 21.1%, respectively), and *Avidekel*^{MR} (16.5% and 20.6%, respectively). Improvements in appetite, with 302 total responses, were attributed to *Midnight*^{MR} (24.8%), *Cognitiva*^{MR} (24.2%), and *Sedamen*^{MR} (22.8%). For improvements in concentration, responses from 191 patients indicate that *Cognitiva*^{MR} (22.0%), *Midnight*^{MR} (20.4%), and *Avidekel*^{MR} (19.4%) were perceived to be the most beneficial strains.

Table 6. Top 10 strains associated with pain improvement at 4-month follow-up and 10-month follow-up

4-months		10-months	
Strain	**n (%)**	**Strain**	**n (%)**
Midnight^{MR}	71 (27.4%)	*Sedamen*^{MR}	40 (29.0%)
Sedamen^{MR}	59 (22.8%)	*Luminarium*^{MR}	36 (26.1%)
Avidekel^{MR}	58 (22.4%)	*Midnight*^{MR}	36 (26.1%)
Luminarium^{MR}	46 (17.8%)	*Avidekel*^{MR}	34 (24.6%)
Cognitiva^{MR}	45 (17.4%)	*Remissio*^{MR}	22 (15.9%)
Eran Almog^{MR}	39 (15.1%)	*Cognitiva*^{MR}	22 (15.9%)
Stellio^{MR}	35 (13.5%)	*Eran Almog*^{MR}	22 (15.9%)
Alaska^{MR}	30 (11.6%)	*Alaska*^{MR}	21 (15.2%)
Bellis^{MR}	24 (9.3%)	*Cerebri*^{MR}	20 (14.5%)
Remissio^{MR}	20 (7.7%)	*Stellio*^{MR}	19 (13.8%)
Total n	259	Total n	138

Improvements in pain as a symptom at 4 months and 10 months

At four months, 259 patients reported on the cannabis varieties that they perceived had caused the greatest reduction in pain levels (see Table 6). A majority of these patients identified *Midnight*^{MR} (27.4%) as the most helpful, followed by *Sedamen*^{MR} (22.8%), and *Avidekel*^{MR} (22.4%). Of the 138 patients who also reported improvement in pain in the 10-month follow-up, most attributed their pain reduction to the variety *Sedamen*^{MR} (29.0%), followed by *Luminarium*^{MR} (26.1%) and *Midnight*^{MR} (26.1%).

DISCUSSION

Different medical cannabis varieties were found to have varying efficacies for the management of different symptoms or conditions. For example, *Eran Amog*^{MR} (very *indica*-dominant, 25-28% THC, 0% CBD, \$15.00/g) was the strain most beneficial for insomnia and sleep disorder, but was the ninth most popular strain overall, and did not appear in the top three varieties for the management of any other condition, symptom, or QOL measure. Similarly, *Stellio*^{MR} was identified as the most beneficial for PTSD and exhaustion, but was reported to be the 14th most effective for overall health, and did not appear to be associated with any other common conditions or symptoms.

On the other hand, several varieties such as *Avidekel*^{MR} and *Midnight*^{MR} were found to be effective across a range of conditions and symptoms. Both varieties contain high CBD content (*Midnight*^{MR} 11-14% CBD, *Avidekel*^{MR} 15-18% CBD), with *Midnight*^{MR} also containing moderate levels of THC (*Midnight*^{MR} 8-11% THC, *Avidekel*^{MR} 0.1-0.8% THC). These two varieties often appeared together as two of the top three strains perceived to be most effective for multiple indications including anxiety disorder, arthritis, sleep problems, and headache. Moreover, *Midnight*^{MR} and *Avidekel*^{MR} both appeared as the top strains for improvements in three out of five QOL items including sleep, concentration, and bowel activity. In these QOL categories, *Midnight*^{MR} was always found to be preferred over *Avidekel*^{MR}. This suggests that a combination of CBD and THC may be more clinically useful than THC or CBD on their own.

Reported improvements in pain 4 and 10 months after intake was remarkably consistent, with the varieties *Midnight*^{MR}, *Sedamen*^{MR}, *Avidekel*^{MR}, and *Luminarium*^{MR} identified as the top four strains by patients at both follow-up intervals. This suggests that these strains may be optimal for pain management. In particular, *Midnight*^{MR} and *Avidekel*^{MR} are likely to contribute to pain reduction in this population due to the anti-inflammatory effects associated with CBD (9). Further investigation should be conducted to determine the optimal CBD:THC ratio for moderating pain in different patient populations. It is also unclear if the efficacy of specific varieties changes over time, and whether they are effective for long-term pain management, past 10-months.

An interaction between CBD and THC has been observed in many physiological studies. For example, studies in mice have found that CBD alters the effect of THC on the protein expression of neurons in multiple brain regions. This is complicated by the fact that the characteristics of CBD-THC interactions vary between different brain regions. In some areas such as the hypothalamus, CBD exerts an antagonistic effect, while in other areas such as the locomotor regions, the effect is synergistic (18). These factors likely play a role in the varying efficacies of different cannabis varieties, and support the finding that varieties containing both CBD and THC may be optimal for many different types of symptom management, as opposed to varieties containing solely CBD or THC.

One of the limitations of this study includes the lack of ability to correlate reported responses of cannabis varieties tried, to patients' actual ordering history from their provider(s). This, in addition to extended follow-up periods, may have led to some level of recall bias influencing results. Improvements in condition or symptoms could also be due to the combination of strains patients tried, making it difficult to accurately attribute any changes in their symptoms or conditions to one isolated product. Moreover, patients' product selection may have been influenced by factors such as differences in strain availability and cannabis variety price.

CONCLUSION

The most frequently reported cannabis strains effective for managing commonly reported conditions or symptoms such as depression, anxiety disorder, and pain include *Midnight^{MR}*, *Luminarium^{MR}*, and *Sedamen^{MR}*.

Strains with high CBD content such as *Avidekel*[MR] and *Midnight*[MR] were effective, particularly for improving pain. These are just a few out of numerous medical cannabis varieties that are available for patients to choose from in the Canadian medical cannabis market. Despite this, limited quality scientific evidence exists to help patients and clinicians with appropriate strain selection. By identifying patient-perceived efficacies of different cannabis varieties, this study provides a platform for clinicians to make accurate strain recommendations to patients presenting a variety of symptoms for which cannabis may be indicated. These results will also help contribute to the strategic design of future efficacy studies.

ACKNOWLEDGMENTS

We thank the generous support of Bratty Family Fund, Michael and Karyn Goldstein Cancer Research Fund, Joey and Mary Furfari Cancer Research Fund, Pulenzas Cancer Research Fund, Joseph and Silvana Melara Cancer Research Fund, and Ofelia Cancer Research Fund. This study was conducted in collaboration with MedReleaf.

REFERENCES

[1]   ElSohly MA, Slade D. Chemical constituents of marijuana: The complex mixture of natural cannabinoids. Life Sci 2005;78(5):539–48.

[2]   Grotenhermen F. The cannabinoid system-a brief review. J Ind Hemp 2004;9(2):87–92.

[3]   Ben Amar M. Cannabinoids in medicine: A review of their therapeutic potential. J Ethnopharmacol 2006;105(1–2):1–25.

[4]   Huestis MA. Human Cannabinoid Pharmacokinetics. Chem Biodivers 2007;4(8):1770–804.

[5]   Whiting PF, Wolff RF, Deshpande S, Di Nisio M, Duffy S, Hernandez A V, et al. Cannabinoids for Medical Use. JAMA 2015;313(24):2456–73.

[6]   Huang W-J, Chen W-W, Zhang X. Endocannabinoid system: Role in depression, reward and pain control (Review). Mol Med Rep 2016;14:2899–903.

[7]   Grotenhermen F, Müller-Vahl K. The Therapeutic Potential of Cannabis and Cannabinoid. Dtsch Arztebl Int 2012;109(29–30):495–501.

[8]   Hill K. Medical Marijuana for Treatment of Chronic Pain and Other Medical and Psychiatric Problems. JAMA 2015;313(24):2474–83.

[9]   Zhornitsky S, Potvin S. Cannabidiol in Humans—The Quest for Therapeutic Targets. Pharmaceuticals 2012;5:529–52.

[10]   F. G. Clinical pharmacodynamics of cannabinoids. J Cannabis Ther 2004;4(1):29–78.

[11]   Szaflarski JP, Martina Bebin E. Cannabis, cannabidiol, and epilepsy - From receptors to clinical response. Epilepsy Behav 2014;41:277–82.

[12]   Russo EB. Taming THC: potential entourage effects. Br J Pharmacol 2011;163:1344–64.

[13]   Hazekamp A, Tejkalová K, Papadimitriou S. Cannabis: From Cultivar to Chemovar II—A metabolomics approach to cannabis classification. Cannabis Cannabinoid Res 2016;1(1):202–15.

[14]   Hazekamp A, Fischedick JT. Cannabis - from cultivar to chemovar. Drug Test Anal 2012;4:660–7.

[15]   Nicholas MK. The pain self-efficacy questionnaire: Taking pain into account. Eur J Pain 11(2):153–63.

[16]   Burckhardt CS, Anderson KL. The Quality of Life Scale (QOLS): reliability, validity, and utilization. Health Qual Life Outcomes 2003;1(60):1–7.

[17]   Fletcher A, Gore S, Jones D, Fitzpatrick R, Spiegelhalter D, Cox D. Quality of life measures in health care. II: Design, analysis, and interpretation. BMJ 1992;305(7):1145–8.

[18]   Todd SM, Arnold JC. Neural correlates of interactions between cannabidiol and Δ(9)-tetrahydrocannabinol in mice: implications for medical cannabis. Br J Pharmacol 2016;173(1):53–65.

In: Medical Cannabis   ISBN: 978-1-53611-907-7
Editors: S. O'Hearn, A. Blake et al. © 2017 Nova Science Publishers, Inc.

Chapter 7

MEDICAL CANNABIS USE FOR PATIENTS WITH POST-TRAUMATIC STRESS DISORDER (PTSD)

Stephanie Chan[1], BSc(C), Alexia Blake[2], MSc,
Amiti Wolt[2], BA, Bo Angela Wan[1], MPhil,
Pearl Zaki[1], BSc(C), Liying Zhang[1], PhD,
Henry Lam[1], MLS, Marissa Slaven[3], MD,
Erynn Shaw[3], MD, Carlo DeAngelis[1], PharmD,
Vithusha Ganesh[1], BSc(C), Leila Malek[1], BSc(Hons),
Edward Chow[1], MBBS and Shannon O'Hearn[2,*], MSc
[1]Odette Cancer Centre, Sunnybrook Health Sciences Centre,
University of Toronto, Toronto, Ontario, Canada
[2]MedReleaf, Markham, Ontario, Canada
[3]Juravinski Cancer Centre, Hamilton Health Sciences,
Hamilton, Ontario, Canada

---

* Correspondence: Ms Shannon O'Hearn MSc, MedReleaf, Markham Industrial Park, Markham
ON, Canada. Email: sohearn@medreleaf.com.

Common symptoms associated with post-traumatic stress disorder (PTSD) include re-experiencing and avoiding trauma-related situations, negative cognitions and mood, and arousal. Early clinical research studies have shown that medical cannabis may minimize these debilitating symptoms. In this chapter we analyzed patient-reported outcomes in patients using medical cannabis for PTSD in Canada. A voluntary online survey was completed by PTSD patients using medical cannabis at baseline, 4-months, and 10-months after initiating use of cannabis from a single medical cannabis provider. Patients reported on outcomes including present symptoms and medical conditions, quality of life (QOL), and side effects experienced from cannabis use. A total of 588 patients with PTSD, predominantly Caucasian (84.4%) males (77.7%) with an average age of 43 years, completed the survey at baseline. There were 58.3% and 48.3% of PTSD patients that reported also having depression and anxiety disorders, respectively. Seventy-eight of 139 (56.1%) patients reported experiencing severe pain at baseline, compared to only 15 (10.8%) patients after 4-months (p<0.0001). Significant improvements were also seen in patients' ability to cope with pain after 4 and 10 months of cannabis use (n=100, p<0.0001). Patients reported significant improvements in overall QOL (n=39, p=0.03) and general mood (n=37, p=0.0005), as well as experience with sleep (n=31, p=0.002) and concentration (n=30, p=0.006) after 4 and 10 months. Patients suffering from PTSD reported significant improvements in a variety symptoms and QOL indicators after 4 months of cannabis use. Cannabis use in this population should be further studied and considered as an alternative treatment option.

INTRODUCTION

Post-traumatic stress disorder (PTSD) is a debilitating trauma and stressor-related disorder that may occur after directly experiencing or witnessing a traumatic event(s) (1). The four symptom cluster domains outlined in the Diagnostic and Statistical Manual of Mental Disorders 5th Edition (DSM-5) are re-experiencing, avoidance, negative cognitions and mood, and arousal (1). Re-experiencing may occur in the form of flashbacks, dreams, or psychological distress pertaining to the traumatic event(s), while avoidance symptoms involve avoiding memories, thoughts, or physical reminders of the event(s). Negative cognition and mood pertains to a variety of emotions such as a distorted sense of blame of others or oneself for the traumatic event(s), or a sense of estrangement or surrealism from others or surroundings. Finally, arousal symptoms may manifest in the form of aggressive and reckless behaviour or hypervigilance and sleep-related problems (1).

Reported rates of exposure to a traumatic event(s) in an individual's lifetime have ranged from 39.1% to 89.6% in the United States (2, 3). In Canada, a study conducted by telephone survey of 2991 individuals in a nationally representative sample reported that 76.1% of participants had exposure to at least one traumatic event sufficient to cause PTSD (4).

In the United States, the lifetime prevalence of PTSD in adults was estimated to be 6.8% according to the National Comorbidity Survey Replication conducted between 2001 and 2002 (5). The lifetime prevalence was 3.6% and 9.7% among men and women, respectively (5). In another study conducted in a sample of 1002 individuals in Winnipeg, Manitoba, the 1-month prevalence of PTSD was found to be 1.2% in men and 8.2% in women (6). Of 3062 surveyed women in Ontario, a 10.7% lifetime prevalence of PTSD was observed (7). In a nationally representative sample of 2991 Canadian individuals, the lifetime and 1-month prevalence of PTSD was estimated to be 9.2% and 2.4%, respectively (4).

PTSD is associated with several behavioural and mental comorbid conditions. In particular, major depressive disorder (MDD), anxiety disorders, and alcohol and substance abuse/dependence are the most common comorbidities (8–10). In Canada, it has been reported that 74% of PTSD patients also suffered from MDD, 27.8% from alcohol abuse/dependence, and 25.5% from substance abuse/dependence (4).

A variety of psychotherapies may be used to treat PTSD including Prolonged Exposure Therapy and Cognitive Processing Therapy. Pharmacological interventions can reduce PTSD symptoms through the modulation of neurotransmitter activity, particularly the activity of serotonin, norepinephrine, gamma-aminobutyric acid, and dopamine. Selective serotonin reuptake inhibitors are generally used as first-line treatment for PTSD, but other antidepressants, mood stabilizers, atypical antipsychotics, tricyclic antidepressants, monoamine oxidase inhibitors or benzodiazepines may also be used (11).

The mammalian endocannabinoid system contains series of receptors known as cannabinoid receptors 1 and 2 (CB-1 and CB-2), upon which endogenous cannabinoids such as anandamide naturally act. The activation of these receptors can produce a multitude of effects including muscle relaxation, pain reduction, appetite stimulation, and the modulation of mood and memory (12). Medical cannabis has shown potential in managing various symptoms of PTSD, predominantly through the interaction of the cannabinoids cannabidiol (CBD) and tetrahydrocannabinol (THC), with the endocannabinoid system. Further, PTSD patients have been reported to have abnormalities in CB-1 receptors and low levels of the endocannabinoid anandamide (13). Therefore, increasing stimulation of the CB-1 pathway with the use of medical cannabis may have potential as an effective treatment option for reducing PTSD-related symptoms in these patients. However, there are very few studies in the literature reporting the efficacy of cannabis in PTSD symptom management (14).

OUR PROJECT

Patients using medical cannabis were invited to complete a voluntary online survey at baseline, prior to initiating treatment with cannabis from the medical cannabis provider. Patients who completed the baseline survey were sent a follow-up (FU) survey 4 months later, which was customized based on their initial baseline responses. Another FU survey was sent to patients 10 months following the completion of the baseline survey if they completed a FU survey at 4 months.

The baseline and follow-up survey consisted of over 100 questions; however, the survey was dynamic and customized to only ask patients questions that were relevant to them (e.g., patients were not asked to answer pain-related questions if they had not experienced any pain at baseline). Therefore, not all patients answered all questions. Patients could also skip questions if they did not want to answer them. The survey was designed to take between 15 and 25 minutes to complete.

Questions were developed based on consultation with nurses and physicians who have experience prescribing medical cannabis to patients, and relevant scientific literature. However, due to the range of patients included and scope of information intended to be collected in this survey, questions were adapted from the literature to be shorter and cover certain parameters in less detail than commonly referenced validated questionnaires. The pain scale used was based on the numeric rating scale, a commonly used method of measuring pain severity in patients with chronic pain (15–17). Questions on patients' ability to cope with pain were based on the Pain Self-Efficacy Questionnaire, which emphasizes the importance of understanding patients' perceived ability to cope with pain (18). The dimensions of quality of life (QOL) covered in the survey were based on a number of validated and commonly used QOL assessment tools (19, 20).

The baseline survey collected demographic information including age, sex, ethnicity, and employment status. Patients were asked to indicate whether they suffered from a wide range of conditions including, but not limited to, type and stage of cancer, diabetes, heart disease, anxiety, depression, PTSD, and autism. Patients were also asked to rate the severity of the conditions they reported as mild, moderate, or severe, and to state how many years they have suffered from the condition. Additional FU questions specific to each of the patient's conditions were posed to better characterize patients' experiences with those conditions.

Additionally, based on a large list of symptoms provided, patients were asked to report which symptoms they experienced regularly and the severity of each symptom (mild, moderate, or severe). If patients indicated they had recurring pain at baseline, they were asked to score their pain on a scale from 1-10, where 1 represented dull pain and 10 represented severe pain. They were also asked to rate their ability to cope with pain (very easy, somewhat easy, somewhat difficult, or very difficult).

QOL questions followed, including questions asking patients to rate their overall QOL (very good, good, fair, bad, very bad) and how capable they were of performing their activities of daily living (ADL) (very capable, somewhat capable, somewhat incapable, very incapable, don't know). Additional questions regarding patients' experience with sleep, appetite, concentration, bowel activity, and sexual function (severe difficulty, moderate difficulty, no difficulty, good, very good), and patients' mobility and ability to dress and shower independently (severe, moderate, minimal, or no difficulty) were asked.

Follow-up

FU surveys were sent to patients 4 months after the completion of the baseline survey and for patients that completed the 4-month FU survey, another survey was sent 10 months following the baseline survey. In the FU surveys, patients were first asked to rate the effect of cannabis on their reported condition(s) (significant deterioration, moderate deterioration, slight deterioration, no change, slight improvement, moderate improvement, significant improvement) and then asked how long it took for cannabis to affect their condition(s).

Patients with pain were also asked to score their pain on a scale from 1-10 and to rate their ability to cope with pain after using cannabis (very easy, somewhat easy, somewhat difficult, very difficult). Questions on QOL and symptoms identical to those from baseline were asked. Additionally, questions on side effects of cannabis use including the type, frequency, duration, and intensity were included.

Baseline and FU surveys were completed between January 2015 and December 2016. Only patients that reported having PTSD in the survey were included in this study.

Descriptive analysis was conducted using proportions for categorical variables, and mean (range) for age. The Fisher exact test or the Chi-squared test was used as appropriate to look for significant associations between pain and ability responses, improvement status (improvement, no change, or deterioration), the presence of most common medical conditions, quality of life and symptoms between baseline and follow-up. A paired t-test was used for comparing baseline and follow up pain scores. Two-sided p-value < 0.05 was considered statistically significant. All analyses were conducted using Statistical Analysis Software (SAS version 9.4, Cary, NC).

OUR FINDINGS

At baseline, 2321 people completed the survey, 588 of which reported having PTSD. Most PTSD patients were male (77.7%) and Caucasian (84.4%) with an average age of 43 years. Of 540 PTSD patients who reported how many years they had suffered from PTSD, 48.3% reported less than 10 years, 27.0% reported 10-19 years, and 24.6% reported 20 or more years. The most common comorbidities reported in PTSD patients at baseline were depression (58.3%), anxiety disorders (48.3%), sleep disorders (35.6%), arthritis (23.2%) and migraines (17.0%). Many patients reported having previous experience with cannabis (78.5%) and currently using cannabis at baseline (85.8%); Table 1 summarizes the demographic information of the PTSD patients included in this study.

Pain and ability to cope with pain

Patients who reported experiencing recurring pain were asked to score their pain severity from 1 to 10 at baseline, 4-month FU and 10-month FU. Between baseline and 4-month FU, a significant reduction in the severity of pain was observed (n=139, p<0.0001) from 56.1% patients reporting severe pain (score of 8-10) at baseline to only 10.8% at 4-month FU. Of the 21 patients who completed the question at baseline, 4-month FU, and 10-month FU, 13 patients (61.9%) at baseline, 3 patients (14.3%) at 4-month FU, and 1 patient (4.8%) at 10-month FU reported experiencing severe pain. This again, demonstrated a statistically significant reduction in the severity of pain following cannabis treatment (p<0.0001).

Table 1. PTSD patient demographics

Demographic	n (%)
Gender	
Male	457 (77.72%)
Female	131 (22.28%)
< 10	261 (48.33%)
10 – 19	146 (27.04%)
≥ 20	133 (24.63%)
Ethnicity	
Caucasian	492 (84.39%)
Spanish/Hispanic/Latino	3 (0.51%)
Native Canadian	38 (6.52%)
Black/African American	1 (0.17%)
Asian	5 (0.86%)
Other	44 (7.54%)
Age (years)	
19 - 29	46 (8.07%)
30 - 39	170 (29.82%)
40 - 49	191 (33.51%)
50 - 59	126 (22.11%)
60 - 69	36 (6.32%)
≥ 70	1 (0.18%)
Average (min, max)	43.25 (19, 70)
Other Conditions	
Depression	344 (58.30%)
Anxiety disorder	285 (48.31%)
Sleep disorder	210 (35.59%)
Arthritis	137 (23.22%)
Migraines	101 (17.00%)
Previous experience with cannabis	
Yes	394 (78.49%)
No	71 (14.14%)
Prefer not to answer	37 (7.37%)
Currently on cannabis	
Yes	339 (85.82%)
No	56 (14.18%)

In all three surveys, patients were asked to describe their ability to cope with pain by selecting one of the following categorical responses: very easy, somewhat easy, somewhat difficult, or very difficult. From baseline to 4-month FU, significantly fewer patients responded 'very difficult' (n=48 at baseline, n=3 at 4-month FU; n=100, p<0.0001). Of the 21 patients who answered this question in all three surveys, 13 (61.9%) responded with 'very difficult' at baseline versus zero patients at 4-month and 10-month FU (p<0.0001). Additionally, only 1 (4.8%) patient at baseline responded with 'somewhat easy' in comparison to 15 (71.4%) and 14 (66.7%) patients at 4-month and 10-month FU, respectively. Table 2 summarizes patients' pain scores and ability to deal with pain at all three time-points.

Table 2. Pain response and ability to cope with pain at baseline, 4-month follow-up, and 10-month follow-up

Patients who responded at baseline and 4-month FU			
	Baseline, n (%)	**4-month, n (%)**	**p-value***
Pain level (n=139)			**<0.0001**
Mild (1-4)	10 (7.19%)	57 (41.01%)	
Moderate (5-7)	51 (36.69%)	67 (48.20%)	
Severe (8-10)	78 (56.12%)	15 (10.79%)	
Ability to deal with pain (n=100)			**<0.0001**
Very easy	2 (2.00%)	13 (13.00%)	
Somewhat easy	8 (8.00%)	69 (69.00%)	
Somewhat difficult	42 (42.00%)	15 (15.00%)	
Very difficult	48 (48.00%)	3 (3.00%)	
Patients who responded at baseline, 4-month and 10-month FU			
	Baseline, n (%)	**4-month, n (%)**	**10-month, n (%)**	**p-value**
Pain level (n=21)				**<0.0001**
Mild (1-4)	0 (0.00%)	8 (38.10%)	14 (66.67%)	
Moderate (5-7)	8 (38.10%)	10 (47.62%)	6 (28.57%)	
Severe (8-10)	13 (61.90%)	3 (14.29%)	1 (4.76%)	
Ability to deal with pain (n=21)				**<0.0001**
Very easy	0 (0.00%)	1 (4.76%)	3 (14.29%)	
Somewhat easy	1 (4.76%)	15 (71.43%)	14 (66.67%)	
Somewhat difficult	7 (33.33%)	5 (23.81%)	4 (19.05%)	
Very difficult	13 (61.90%)	0 (0.00%)	0 (0.00%)	

*Bolded p-values are statistically significant.

Improvements in medical conditions

Patients reported changes in other medical conditions from baseline by selecting one of the following categorical responses: significant deterioration, moderate deterioration, slight deterioration, no change, slight improvement, moderate improvement, or significant improvement. At 4-month follow-up, 73.7% (n=56), 78.3% (n=47), 74.0% (n=37), 68.8% (n=22), and 76.9% (n=10) of patients reported an improvement in depression, anxiety disorders, sleep disorders, arthritis, and migraines, respectively (Table 3). Although many patients reported improvements in their conditions, this was not statistically significant.

**Table 3. Improvement in most common medical conditions
at 4-month follow-up**

Condition	Improvement, n (%)	No change, n (%)	Deterioration, n (%)	Total n	p-value
Depression	56 (73.68%)	11 (14.47%)	9 (11.84%)	76	0.7173
Anxiety disorder	47 (78.33)	4 (6.67%)	9 (15.00%)	60	0.9993
Sleep disorder	37 (74.00%)	7 (14.00%)	6 (12.00%)	50	0.8293
Arthritis	22 (68.75%)	5 (15.63%)	5 (15.63%)	32	0.7862
Migraines	10 (76.92%)	2 (15.38%)	1 (7.69%)	13	0.5238

Improvements in quality of life (QOL)

Questions were asked on overall QOL, general mood, mobility, ability to dress and shower independently, and ability to perform activities of daily living (ADLs) (Table 4), in addition to patients' experience with sleep, appetite, concentration, bowel activity, and sexual function (Table 5). From baseline to 4-month and 10-month FU, improvements in all QOL indicators were observed; for the overall QOL item, significantly more patients reported having 'good' or 'very good' overall QOL (n=33, p=0.03) and a 'positive' or 'very positive' mood (n=37, p=0.0005). More patients also reported 'minimal difficulty' or 'no difficulty' in mobility and ability to dress and shower independently (n=36; n=38), and felt 'somewhat capable' or 'very capable' in their ability to perform ADLs (n=39);

however, these were not statistically significant. When asked to describe their experience with several aspects of their QOL, patients were given the following options: severe difficulty, moderate difficulty, no difficulty, good, and very good. Significantly fewer patients had difficulties and more patients used 'good' and 'very good' to describe their experience with sleep (n=31, p=0.002) and concentration (n=30, p=0.006) from baseline to 4-month and 10-month FU. This association was also seen for appetite, bowel activity, and sexual function, but with no statistical significance.

Table 4. Improvement in quality of life at 4-month and 10-month follow-up

	Baseline, n(%)	4-month, n (%)	10-month, n (%)	p-value*
Overall quality of Life (n=39)				**0.0280**
Very good	2 (5.1%)	5 (12.8%)	3 (7.7%)	
Good	2 (5.1%)	9 (23.1%)	13 (33.3%)	
Fair	18 (46.2%)	18 (46.2%)	15 (38.5%)	
Bad	11 (28.2%)	5 (12.8%)	7 (17.9%)	
Very bad	6 (15.4%)	2 (5.1%)	1 (2.6%)	
General mood (n=37)				**0.0005**
Very positive	1 (2.7%)	2 (5.4%)	4 (10.8%)	
Positive	7 (18.9%)	9 (24.3%)	12 (32.4%)	
Neutral	13 (35.1%)	24 (64.9%)	12 (32.4%)	
Negative	14 (37.8%)	0 (0%)	8 (21.6%)	
Very negative	2 (5.4%)	2 (5.4%)	1 (2.7%)	
Mobility (n=36)				**0.3686**
Severe difficulty	5 (13.9%)	4 (11.1%)	4 (11.1%)	
Moderate difficulty	13 (36.1%)	6 (16.7%)	10 (27.8%)	
Minimal difficulty	8 (22.2%)	16 (44.4%)	9 (25%)	
No difficulty	10 (27.8%)	10 (27.8%)	13 (36.1%)	
Ability to dress/shower independently (n=38)				0.9845
Severe difficulty	1 (2.6%)	1 (2.6%)	0 (0%)	
Moderate difficulty	6 (15.8%)	4 (10.5%)	6 (15.8%)	
Minimal difficulty	14 (36.8%)	13 (34.2%)	12 (31.6%)	
No difficulty	17 (44.7%)	20 (52.6%)	20 (52.6%)	
Ability to perform ADLs (n=39)				0.6141
Very capable	12 (30.8%)	9 (23.1%)	11 (28.2%)	
Somewhat capable	12 (30.8%)	19 (48.7%)	16 (41%)	
Somewhat incapable	6 (15.4%)	8 (20.5%)	5 (12.8%)	
Very incapable	8 (20.5%)	3 (7.7%)	6 (15.4%)	
Don't know	1 (2.6%)	0 (0%)	1 (2.6%)	

*Bolded p-values are statistically significant. ADL: activities of daily living.

Table 5. Improvement in experience with sleep, appetite, concentration, bowel activity, and sexual function

Assessment time	Response, n (%)					p-value
	Severe difficulty	Moderate difficulty	No difficulty	Good	Very good	
Sleep (n=34)						**0.0015**
Baseline	19 (54.3%)	14 (40%)	1 (2.9%)	0 (0%)	1 (2.9%)	
4-month	5 (14.3%)	14 (40%)	4 (11.4%)	5 (14.3%)	7 (20%)	
10-month	7 (20%)	15 (42.9%)	2 (5.7%)	6 (17.1%)	5 (14.3%)	
Appetite (n=35)						0.3581
Baseline	6 (16.7%)	11 (30.6%)	8 (22.2%)	10 (27.8%)	1 (2.8%)	
4-month	2 (5.6%)	8 (22.2%)	6 (16.7%)	16 (44.4%)	4 (11.1%)	
10-month	2 (5.6%)	6 (16.7%)	10 (27.8%)	16 (44.4%)	2 (5.6%)	
Concentration (n=34)						**0.0061**
Baseline	14 (40%)	15 (42.9%)	1 (2.9%)	4 (11.4%)	1 (2.9%)	
4-month	2 (5.7%)	16 (45.7%)	4 (11.4%)	8 (22.9%)	5 (14.3%)	
10-month	14 (40%)	15 (42.9%)	1 (2.9%)	4 (11.4%)	1 (2.9%)	
Bowel activity (n=36)						0.1426
Baseline	4 (11.1%)	12 (33.3%)	6 (16.7%)	7 (19.4%)	7 (19.4%)	
4-month	0 (0%)	13 (36.1%)	5 (13.9%)	10 (27.8%)	8 (22.2%)	
10-month	3 (8.3%)	9 (25%)	10 (27.8%)	12 (33.3%)	2 (5.6%)	
Sexual function (n=21)						0.0742
Baseline	11 (32.4%)	6 (17.6%)	7 (20.6%)	2 (5.9%)	8 (23.5%)	
4-month	5 (14.7%)	7 (20.6%)	6 (17.6%)	12 (35.3%)	4 (11.8%)	
10-month	5 (14.7%)	5 (14.7%)	7 (20.6%)	12 (35.3%)	5 (14.7%)	

*Bolded p-values are statistically significant.

Improvements in symptoms

The most commonly reported symptoms in PTSD patients were anxiety, sleep problems, depression, insomnia, exhaustion, and headaches. Table 6 describes the distribution of the severities of these symptoms. At 4-month FU and 10-month FU, patients reported how the severity of these symptoms had changed since baseline by selecting one of the following options: significant deterioration, moderate deterioration, slight deterioration, no change, slight improvement, moderate improvement, significant improvement, or no longer have this symptom (Table 7). In the 4-month FU survey, 64-79% of patients reported improvements in the symptoms they reported experiencing at baseline. At the 10-month FU survey, 73-83% of patients reported improvements in their symptoms compared to baseline. However, only improvements in exhaustion at 4-month FU were statistically significant (p=0.009).

Table 6. Severity of most common symptoms at baseline

Symptom	Mild, n (%)	Moderate, n (%)	Severe, n (%)	Total n
Anxiety	50 (9.1%)	264 (48.2%)	234 (42.7%)	548
Sleep problems	61 (12.0%)	214 (24.0%)	234 (46.0%)	509
Depression	81 (16.4%)	233 (45.0%)	182 (37.0%)	496
Insomnia	59 (13.7%)	191 (44.3%)	181 (42.0%)	431
Exhaustion	76 (20.5%)	189 (50.9%)	106 (28.6%)	371
Headache	131 (37.2%)	149 (42.3%)	72 (20.4%)	352

Table 7. Improvement in most common symptoms from baseline to 4-month and to 10-month follow-up

Symptom	Improvement, n (%)	No change, n (%)	Deterioration, n (%)	Total n	p-value*
4-month FU					
Anxiety	121 (79.1%)	15 (9.8%)	17 (11.1%)	153	0.0962
Sleep problems	104 (75.4%)	19 (13.8%)	15 (10.9%)	138	0.8678
Depression	109 (78.4%)	15 (10.8%)	15 (10.8%)	139	0.2476
Insomnia	82 (73.2%)	20 (17.9%)	10 (8.9%)	112	0.6330
Exhaustion	60 (63.8%)	25 (26.6%)	9 (9.6%)	94	**0.0086**
Headache	54 (67.5%)	16 (20.0%)	10 (12.5%)	80	0.3063
10-month FU					
Anxiety	30 (83.3%)	2 (5.6%)	4 (11.1%)	36	0.2681
Sleep problems	28 (82.4%)	4 (11.8%)	2 (5.9%)	34	0.9752
Depression	28 (82.4%)	4 (11.8%)	2 (5.9%)	34	0.9752
Insomnia	23 (82.1%)	4 (14.3%)	1 (3.6%)	28	0.7862
Exhaustion	16 (72.7%)	4 (18.2%)	2 (9.1%)	22	0.4003
Headache	20 (83.3%)	3 (12.5%)	1 (4.2%)	24	0.8623

*Bolded p-values are statistically significant.

Side effects

Of the 115 patients that answered questions regarding side effects experienced from cannabis use at 4-month FU, the most common side effects were dry mouth (n=22), psycho-active effects (n=15), sleepiness (n=13), red or irritated eyes (n=8), increased heart rate (n=6), and decreased memory (n=7). The severities of these side effects were mostly mild, with no patients reporting severe for red or irritated eyes, increased heart rate, and decreased memory. Table 8 summarizes the severity of these side effects.

Table 8. Most common side effects at 4-month follow-up

Side effect (Total n=115)	Mild, n (%)	Moderate n (%)	Severe, n (%)	Total n
Dry mouth	10 (45.5%)	9 (40.9%)	3 (13.6%)	22
Psycho-active effects (feeling "high")	6 (40.0%)	7 (46.7%)	2 (13.3%)	15
Sleepiness	5 (38.5%)	7 (53.8%)	1 (7.7%)	13
Red/Irritated eyes	6 (75.0%)	2 (25.0%)	0 (0.0%)	8
Heart palpitations (increased heart rate)	5 (83.3%)	1 (16.6%)	0 (0.0%)	6
Decreased memory	6 (85.7%)	1 (14.3%)	0 (0.0%)	7

DISCUSSION

This chapter presents the results of a voluntary online survey administered by a Canadian medical cannabis provider for patients with PTSD.

Few studies have analysed the efficacy of cannabis in reducing symptoms in PTSD patients, and those that have been conducted have shown varying results. A retrospective chart review by Greer et al. (21) of 80 consecutive patients participating in the New Mexico Department of Health's Medical Cannabis Program for PTSD saw an over 75% reduction in all three PTSD symptom clusters as measured by the Clinician

Administered Posttraumatic Scale for DSM-IV (CAPS) when on cannabis compared to off cannabis (21). However, these patients were expected to have significant symptom reduction, as all patients had previous experience with cannabis and had already found that cannabis improved their PTSD symptoms. Therefore, they were entering the program for the purpose of legally obtaining cannabis. As well, patients may have experienced some exaggerated PTSD symptoms when off cannabis due to cannabis-withdrawal syndrome; thus, this study's confounding factors make it difficult to determine the effects of cannabis in the general PTSD population (21). In a study by Fraser (22), nabilone (an orally administered synthetic cannabinoid based drug) use in 47 PTSD patients with a 2-year history of PTSD-related nightmares that were unresponsive to standard treatment resulted in total cessation of nightmares or a reduction in nightmare severity in 72% of patients (22). Roitman et al. conducted an open, pilot study to determine the safety and efficacy of an oral Δ9-tetrahydrocannabinol (THC) as an add-on treatment in PTSD patients in Israel. Of the 10 patients studied, significant reductions in symptom severity were observed in the CAPS hyperarousal symptom cluster as well as sleep quality, frequency of nightmares, and nightmare effects (23). Wilkinson et al. (24) studied 2,276 veterans with PTSD admitted to a Veterans Affairs treatment program. Those who started marijuana use after discharge were associated with significantly worse PTSD symptom severity, more violent behaviour, and more alcohol and drug use compared to those who never used or stopped marijuana use after discharge (24). The present study reports contrasting results, in which after 4 and 10 months of treatment with medical cannabis, PTSD patients reported significant improvements in pain and their ability to cope with pain, as well as medical conditions, QOL, and symptoms.

Dry mouth, psychoactive effects, and sleepiness were the most common side effects of cannabis use reported by PTSD patients in the present study. Of the 10 patients in the open pilot study by Roitman et al. (23), two experienced side effects of dry mouth, one experienced headache, and one experienced dizziness (23). In the study of 47 patients using nabilone for PTSD-related nightmares conducted by Fraser, 13 patients experienced side effects such as light-headedness, forgetfulness, dizziness, and headache resulting in cessation of nabilone therapy (22). Therefore, it is important for physicians prescribing cannabis for PTSD to be aware of possible side effects and to monitor the severity of these side effects closely.

In a study by Bonn-Miller et al. (25), 217 medical cannabis users filled out a series of questionnaires pertaining to cannabis use and efficacy, 18.9% of whom had PTSD and reported cannabis was 'moderately' to 'quite a bit' helpful. However, cannabis abuse and dependence was observed in 22.5% of PTSD patients (25). Bohnert et al. (26) observed that of 186 patients newly referred for medical cannabis, 23% had a lifetime history of PTSD and the PTSD patients had significantly higher lifetime use of prescription opioids, cocaine, prescription sedatives, and street opioids compared to patients without PTSD in the same sample (26). These studies emphasize the importance of closely monitoring substance abuse, alcohol abuse, and specifically, cannabis abuse or dependence in this population.

The present study suffers from several limitations. Firstly, no validated questionnaires pertaining to PTSD symptoms were used such as the PTSD checklist for DSM-5 (PCL-5). Additionally, the compliance rate for the survey was extremely low, which is reflected in the low patient numbers for certain parameters at FU despite the large sample size. This could explain why even though trends indicated improved QOL, many values were not statistically significant. Also, patients were not required to complete the survey at exactly 4 or 10 months following initiation of cannabis use, thus the survey could have been done at any time-point after the survey request had been sent.

The survey administered for the present study was also unable to account for other pain medications or study adverse events or hospitalization occurring during treatment. Additionally, only 1516 of the 2,321 patients (including non-PTSD patients) that initially completed the survey were invited for a follow-up survey. Some patients had not reached the 4-month point after starting cannabis use (n=552), while 253 patients either stopped medical cannabis treatment or switched providers. Of the

1,516 active patients invited for a follow-up survey, it is uncertain whether these patients were actively taking cannabis. However, it is very likely that they were, based on their active prescriptions with the cannabis provider as well as the fact that they took the time to complete the survey. As the survey is voluntary, it is possible that patients who had a positive experience with medical cannabis were more likely to fill the survey, resulting in a skew towards positive responses in our results. Finally, at baseline, around 86% of patients responded with 'yes' when asked if they were currently consuming cannabis, meaning that the improvements in symptoms and QOL observed may reflect switching cannabis treatment rather than the efficacy of cannabis in general.

CONCLUSION

The present study observed significant improvements in PTSD symptoms and QOL in a sample of Canadian PTSD patients after using medical cannabis. Further investigations are required regarding the safety and efficacy of medical cannabis in this patient population. Clinical trials are recommended to determine whether medical cannabis is an appropriate alternative treatment option for symptom relief in PTSD patients.

ACKNOWLEDGMENTS

We thank the generous support of Bratty Family Fund, Michael and Karyn Goldstein Cancer Research Fund, Joey and Mary Furfari Cancer Research Fund, Pulenzas Cancer Research Fund, Joseph and Silvana Melara Cancer Research Fund, and Ofelia Cancer Research Fund. This study was conducted in collaboration with MedReleaf.

REFERENCES

[1]   American Psychiatric Association. Trauma- and stressor-related disorders. In: Diagnostic and statistical manual of mental disorders, Fifth edition. Arlington, VA: American Psychiatric Association, 2013.

[2]   Breslau N, Davis GC, Andreski P, Peterson E. Traumatic events and posttraumatic stress disorder in an urban population of young adults. Arch Gen Psychiatry 1991;48(3):216–22.

[3]   Breslau N, Kessler RC, Chilcoat HD, Schultz LR, Davis GC, Andreski P. Trauma and posttraumatic stress disorder in the community: the 1996 Detroit area survey of trauma. Arch Gen Psychiatry 1998;55(7):626–32.

[4]   Van Ameringen M, Mancini C, Patterson B, Boyle MH. Post-traumatic stress disorder in Canada. CNS Neurosci Ther 2008;14(3):171–81.

[5]   Harvard Medical School. National Comorbidity Survey (NCS), 2005 URL: http://www.hcp.med.harvard.edu.myaccess.library.utoronto.ca/ncs/.

[6]   Stein MB, Walker JR, Forde DR. Gender differences in susceptibility to posttraumatic stress disorder. Behav Res Ther 2000;38(6):619–28.

[7]   Frise S, Steingart A, Sloan M, Cotterchio M, Kreiger N. Psychiatric disorders and use of mental health services by Ontario women. Can J Psychiatry 2002;47(9):849–56.

[8]   Kessler RC, Sonnega A, Bromet E, Hughes M, Nelson CB. Posttraumatic stress disorder in the National Comorbidity Survey. Arch Gen Psychiatry 1995;52(12):1048–60.

[9]   Creamer M, Burgess P, McFarlane AC. Post-traumatic stress disorder: findings from the Australian National Survey of Mental Health and Well-being. Psychol Med 2001;31(7):1237–47.

[10]   Helzer JE, Robins LN, McEvoy L. Post-traumatic stress disorder in the general population. Findings of the epidemiologic catchment area survey. N Engl J Med 1987;317(26):1630–4.

[11]   Jeffreys M. Clinician's Guide to Medications for PTSD, 2016 URL: http://www.ptsd.va.gov/professional/treatment/overview/clinicians-guide-to-medications-for-ptsd.asp.

[12]   Grotenhermen F. The cannabinoid system-a brief review. J Ind Hemp 2004;9(2):87–92.

[13]   Neumeister A, Normandin MD, Pietrzak RH, Piomelli D, Zheng MQ, Gujarro-Anton A, et al. Elevated brain cannabinoid CB1 receptor availability in post-traumatic stress disorder: a positron emission tomography study. Mol Psychiatry 2013;18(9):1034–40.

[14]   Walsh Z, Gonzalez R, Crosby K, S. Thiessen M, Carroll C, Bonn-Miller MO. Medical cannabis and mental health: A guided systematic review. Clin Psychol Rev 2017;51:15–29.

[15]   Krebs EE, Carey TS, Weinberger M. Accuracy of the pain numeric rating scale as a screening test in primary care. J Gen Intern Med 2007;22(10):1453–8.

[16]   Hawker GA, Mian S, Kendzerska T, French M. Measures of adult pain: Visual Analog Scale for Pain (VAS Pain), Numeric Rating Scale for Pain (NRS Pain), McGill Pain Questionnaire (MPQ), Short-Form McGill Pain Questionnaire (SF-MPQ), Chronic Pain Grade Scale (CPGS), Short Form-36 Bodily Pain Scale (SF-36). Arthritis Care Res (Hoboken) 2011;63(S11):S240–52.

[17]   Farrar JT, Young JP, LaMoreaux L, Werth JL, Poole RM. Clinical importance of changes in chronic pain intensity measured on an 11-point numerical pain rating scale. Pain 2001;94(2):149–58.

[18]   Nicholas MK. The pain self-efficacy questionnaire: Taking pain into account. Eur J Pain 2007;11(2):153–63.

[19]   Burckhardt CS, Anderson KL. The Quality of Life Scale (QOLS): reliability, validity, and utilization. Health Qual Life Outcomes 2003;1:60.

[20]   Fletcher A, Gore S, Jones D, Fitzpatrick R, Spiegelhalter D, Cox D. Quality of life measures in health care. II: Design, analysis, and interpretation. BMJ 1992;305(6862):1145-8.

[21]   Greer GR, Grob CS, Halberstadt AL. PTSD symptom reports of patients evaluated for the New Mexico Medical Cannabis Program. J Psychoactive Drugs 2014;46(1):73–7.

[22]   Fraser GA. The use of a synthetic cannabinoid in the management of treatment-resistant nightmares in posttraumatic stress disorder (PTSD). CNS Neurosci Ther 2009;15(1):84–8.

[23]   Roitman P, Mechoulam R, Cooper-Kazaz R, Shalev A. Preliminary, open-label, pilot study of add-on oral Δ9-tetrahydrocannabinol in chronic post-traumatic stress disorder. Clin Drug Investig 2014;34(8):587–91.

[24]   Wilkinson ST, Stefanovics E, Rosenheck RA. Marijuana use is associated with worse outcomes in symptom severity and violent behavior in patients with posttraumatic stress disorder. J Clin Psychiatry 2015;1174–80.

[25]   Bonn-Miller MO, Boden MT, Bucossi MM, Babson KA. Self-reported cannabis use characteristics, patterns and helpfulness among medical cannabis users. Am J Drug Alcohol Abuse 2014;40(1):23–30.

[26]   Bohnert KM, Perron BE, Ashrafioun L, Kleinberg F, Jannausch M, Ilgen MA. Positive posttraumatic stress disorder screens among first-time medical cannabis patients: Prevalence and association with other substance use. Addict Behav 2014;39(10):1414–7.

In: Medical Cannabis   ISBN: 978-1-53611-907-7
Editors: S. O'Hearn, A. Blake et al. © 2017 Nova Science Publishers, Inc.

Chapter 8

MEDICAL CANNABIS USE IN MILITARY AND POLICE VETERANS DIAGNOSED WITH POST-TRAUMATIC STRESS DISORDER (PTSD)

Paul A Smith[1], MD, Stephanie Chan[2], BSc(C),
Alexia Blake[3], MSc, Amiti Wolt[3], BA,
Liying Zhang[2], PhD, Bo Angela Wan[2], MPhil,
Pearl Zaki[2], BSc(C), Henry Lam[2], MLS,
Carlo DeAngelis[2], PharmD, Marissa Slaven[4], MD,
Erynn Shaw[4], MD, Vithusha Ganesh[2], BSc(C),
Leila Malek[1], BSc(Hons), Edward Chow[2], MBBS
and Shannon O'Hearn[3,], MSc*

[1]Dr Paul Smith Professional Corporation, Fredericton, New Brunswick,
[2]Odette Cancer Centre, Sunnybrook Health Sciences Centre, University
of Toronto, Toronto, Ontario
[3]MedReleaf, Markham, Ontario, Canada
[4]Juravinski Cancer Centre, Hamilton Health Sciences, Hamilton,
Ontario, Canada

---

[*] Correspondence: Ms Shannon O'Hearn MSc, MedReleaf Corp, Markham Industrial Park, Markham ON, Canada. Email: sohearn@medreleaf.com.

Post-traumatic stress disorder (PTSD) is a mental illness with intrusive symptoms related to a traumatic event(s), usually treated with pharmacotherapy and psychotherapy. In this chapter, we wanted to assess outcomes in military and police veterans with PTSD treated with medical cannabis, through a retrospective chart review. Veterans with PTSD using medical cannabis after unsuccessful pharmacotherapy and psychotherapy treatment were assessed in a single centre review at baseline and follow-up. Changes in outcomes and PTSD medications from baseline to follow-up were reported with percent change and effect size (ES) and then compared to the minimal clinically important difference. A total of 100 patients (97% male, average age 43 years old) were assessed from January 2014 to January 2016. The aggregate score of PTSD symptoms was reduced from a mean score of 7.0 at baseline to 2.9 at follow-up (59% reduction, ES 1.5, very large effect; $p < 0.0001$). Suicidal thoughts decreased from 4.1 to 0.9 (77% reduction, ES 1.0, large effect; $p<0.0001$). The aggregate score for the impact of PTSD on social and family life was reduced from 6.6 to 2.7 (59% reduction, ES 1.2, large effect; $p<0.0001$). Pain severity decreased from an average of 6.6 to 3.4 (48% reduction, ES 1.5, very large effect). Consumption of PTSD-related medications reduced by 50% from baseline to follow-up. Treatment with medical cannabis in military and police veterans with PTSD who had failed conventional therapy resulted in significant improvements across all PTSD symptoms, as well as social and family impact outcomes and pain severity.

INTRODUCTION

Post-traumatic stress disorder (PTSD) is a mental illness originating from experiencing or witnessing a severe traumatic event(s), resulting in debilitating symptoms in each of the four symptom clusters defined by the "Diagnostic and statistical manual of mental disorders, 5th Edition" (DSM-5). These symptom clusters include re-experiencing, avoidance, negative cognitions and mood, and arousal, and persist longer than one month, causing social or occupational impairment (1). In a study by Rapaport et al. (2), 59% of PTSD patients were found to have clinically severe impairment in quality of life (QOL) (defined by two or more standard deviations under the community norm), even more so than patients with panic disorder (20%), obsessive compulsive disorder (26%), and social phobia (21%) (2).

In Canada, a telephone survey of a nationally representative sample of 2991 patients revealed that 76.1% of participants had been exposed to one or more traumatic events that could potentially cause PTSD (3). This same study found the lifetime prevalence of PTSD to be 9.2% and the 1-month prevalence to be 2.4% (3). In a study of 1002 participants from Winnipeg, Manitoba, the 1-month prevalence of full or partial PTSD was 1.2% and 8.2% in men and women, respectively (4). A lifetime prevalence of PTSD of 10.7% was observed in a sample of 3062 Ontario women (5).

Amongst war veterans, the prevalence of PTSD is higher than in the civilian population. In a literature review related to mental health in the Canadian Armed Forces, the point prevalence of PTSD ranged from 2.1% to 8.1%, and 12-month prevalence was reported at 2.8% (6). Over a 4-year follow-up, studies reported 8% to 20% of Canadian Forces veterans were diagnosed with PTSD at some point in their lives (6).

PTSD is conventionally treated with pharmacotherapy and psychotherapy. Traditional pharmacotherapy for PTSD includes selective serotonin reuptake inhibitors (SSRIs), tricyclic antidepressants, adrenoceptor agonists or antagonists, anticonvulsants, antipsychotics and monoamine oxidase inhibitors (MAOIs) (7). However, findings from pharmacotherapy trials on patient populations with combat-related PTSD, which tends to be more chronic or severe, have been inconsistent and less effective compared to civilian PTSD (8–15). For instance, one double-blind, placebo controlled trial investigating SSRI efficacy in combat-related PTSD saw only a 25-33% reduction in PTSD symptom clusters (16), compared to 40-53% in civilian PTSD, although the combat-related PTSD patients had more severe symptoms at baseline (17, 18). Additionally, a study by van der Kolk et al. saw that PTSD patients using fluoxetine (an SSRI used to treat PTSD) had significantly improved PTSD symptoms compared to patients on a placebo after 5 weeks (n=64) (15). However, a study by Hertzberg et al. also conducted to establish the efficacy of fluoxetine in treating PTSD reported that patients with combat-related PTSD did not have improved PTSD symptomatology when using fluoxetine compared to a placebo (n=12) (14).

Recently, medical cannabis has emerged as a potential alternative treatment option for managing PTSD symptoms when traditional methods are unsuccessful. However, the current literature lacks strong evidence demonstrating the efficacy of medical cannabis within this patient group (19,20). The objective of this chapter was to assess if medical cannabis improved the quality of life and reduced PTSD-related symptoms in Canadian military and police veterans with PTSD through a retrospective chart review.

OUR STUDY

The present study was a retrospective chart audit conducted at a single medical practice experienced in treating military veterans diagnosed with PTSD. 100 consecutive veteran patients who had begun cannabis treatment were assessed. These patients were initially referred to the clinic by the physician(s) managing their prior treatment after failing both pharmacotherapy and psychotherapy. Patients were included in the present review if they had a confirmed diagnosis of PTSD, were military or police veterans, and initiated the use of medical cannabis between January 2014 to January 2016. Patients were started on a dose of 1 gram/day, and self-titrated until desired results were met with instructions of a ceiling dose of 10 grams/day.

Patient charts were retrospectively reviewed by a single individual to assess data collected prior to initiation of medical cannabis treatment, referred to as baseline, and at the first follow-up visit.

At baseline, demographic information including age, gender, marital status, employment status, length of military or police service, alcohol and tobacco use, family history of medical conditions, and patient's history of medical conditions was reviewed. Additionally, patient reported pain severity, measured on a scale of 0 to 10, with 10 being the worst possible pain was assessed. Current medication use and dosages were extracted, if available.

In the patient charts, the severities of several PTSD-related symptoms were scored on a scale of 0 to 10, with 10 being the most severe. These symptoms include danger and irritability, anxiety, avoidance of trigger-related people and situations, depression, distorted sense of blame for events, easily startled, depersonalization, flashbacks or intrusive memories, hyper-vigilance, nightmares, poor concentration, sense that one's surroundings are not real, severe emotional state, and suicidal thoughts. Patients were also asked to rate how PTSD affected their social and family life, including drug and alcohol overuse, marital/relationship harmony, relationship with siblings and parents, and several religious or personal beliefs on a scale from 0 to 10, where 10 indicated an extremely negative effect. Finally, the efficacy of other attempted treatments was recorded using a scale from 0 to 10, with 10 representing the most success.

At follow-up, data on dose and strains of medical cannabis used, and the method of administration was recorded. In addition, current medications, alcohol and tobacco use, pain severity, PTSD symptoms, previous treatments, and effect of PTSD on social and family life were also documented in patient charts. These outcomes were compared to those collected at baseline.

Changes in the average score for each outcome across all participants from baseline to follow-up were analyzed. For each outcome, responses were included in the average only if patients had information available at both the baseline and follow-up. The percentage change in the average score of each outcome and magnitude of effect as measured by effect size (ES) was calculated. Effect size is a quantitative measure of how strong the differences between average outcomes at baseline and follow-up are. An ES of 0.8 to 1.29 was considered large, and an ES of 1.3 or higher was very large. ES was calculated using Cohen's term d (21). Paired t-test was also used to compare baseline and follow-up scores for each outcome. A p-value < 0.05 was considered statistically significant.

The minimal clinically important difference (MCID) is the minimal change associated with a significant benefit from a clinical perspective, rather than a statistical perspective. The MCID was calculated for each outcome and changes from baseline to follow-up were compared against the corresponding MCID (22).

Changes in other PTSD related medications used were detailed in terms of average number of PTSD-related medications and percent change for patients with information available at both baseline and follow-up. Medications considered related to PTSD include medications for pain, depression, anti-psychotic medications, medications for bipolar disorder, anxiety, ADHD, seizures, muscle relaxants, nightmares, sleep and related effects, such as erectile dysfunction and nausea.

This study did not capture details of adverse events, hospitalization, or other physician visits that occurred while using medical cannabis. All analyses were conducted using Statistical Analysis Software (SAS version 9.4 for Windows, Cary, NC).

FINDINGS

A total of 100 patients were assessed. They were primarily male (97%) and on average 43 years old. Two-thirds of patients were unable to work or had retired (see Table 1).

Table 1. Demographic Information (n=100)

Demographics	n (%)
Average age (years)	43
Male	97 (97%)
Age distribution	
<40 years	34 (34%)
40-49 years	41 (41%)
50-59 years	21 (21%)
60+ years	4 (4%)
Employment status at time of baseline visit	
Working	21 (21%)
Student	2 (2%)
Retired/unable to work	63 (63%)
Unknown	14 (14%)

Table 2. Time to follow-up (n=100)

Distribution of time to follow-up visit	n (%)
≤ 3 months	25 (25%)
4-6 months	12 (12%)
7-10 months	11 (11%)
11-12 months	25 (25%)
13-15 months	20 (20%)
16-18 months	7 (7%)

Table 3. Dose of medical cannabis at follow-up (n=99)

Dose of medical cannabis	n (%)
<5 grams	5 (5%)
5 to 9 grams	20 (20%)
10 grams	66 (67%)
More than 10 grams	8 (8%)

Table 4. Composition of medical cannabis varieties

Variety name	THC%	CBD%	Composition
Avidekel[MR]	0.1 - 0.8	15 - 18	*sativa*-leaning
Midnight[MR]	8 - 11	11 - 14	*indica*-leaning
Sedamen[MR"]	21 - 24	0	*indica*-dominant
Luminarium[MR]	25 - 28	0	*sativa*-dominant

THC: tetrahydrocannabinol.
CBD: cannabidiol.

Results collected at baseline were compared to those obtained at follow-up for each scored outcome. Time to follow-up ranged from less than 3 months to 18 months, with follow-up occurring most commonly less than 3 months or 11-12 months after baseline. Table 2 shows the distribution of time to follow-up. Patients were taking 9.4 grams of medical cannabis per day on average at follow-up. Table 3 shows the distribution of doses of medical cannabis used at follow-up. Many varieties of medical cannabis were used by these patients including *Luminarium*[MR], *Sedamen*[MR"], *Midnight*[MR], *Avidekel*[MR] and others supplied by MedReleaf

Corp. Patients were often using multiple strains simultaneously with varying cannabidiol (CBD) and tetrahydrocannabinol (THC) content. Table 4 summarizes the strain composition of several medical cannabis varieties used by patients.

Table 5. Severity of symptoms at baseline and follow-up (Scale of 0-10)

Symptom	Number of responses	Mean baseline score ± SD	Mean follow-up Score ± SD	Improvement (%)	Effect size	p-value*
Anger and irritability	93	7.9 ± 2.1	3.0 ± 2.1	5.0 (63%)	2.4	<.0001
Anxiety	93	7.8 ± 1.5	3.3 ± 1.5	4.6 (59%)	9.0	<.0001
Avoidance of trigger related people and situations	90	8.1 ± 2.3	3.7 ± 2.3	4.3 (54%)	1.9	<.0001
Depression	92	7.3 ± 2.1	2.9 ± 2.1	4.4 (60%)	2.1	<.0001
Distorted sense of blame for the events	78	6.7 ± 2.8	2.9 ± 2.8	3.8 (57%)	1.4	<.0001
Easily startled	90	7.5 ± 2.3	3.3 ± 2.3	4.2 (57%)	1.8	<.0001
Feeling disconnected from oneself (depersonalization)	78	7.0 ± 2.7	2.5 ±2.7	4.4 (64%)	1.6	<.0001
Flashbacks and intrusive memories	89	6.9 ± 2.4	2.8 ±2.4	4.2 (60%)	1.7	<.0001
Hyper-vigilance	84	7.4 ± 2.2	3.0 ± 2.2	4.4 (59%)	2.0	<.0001
Nightmares	87	6.8 ± 2.5	2.5 ± 2.5	4.2 (62%)	1.7	<.0001
Poor concentration	92	8.0 ± 1.8	4.2 ± 1.8	3.8 (47%)	2.0	<.0001
Sense or feeling that one's surroundings are not real	76	4.8 ± 3.4	1.9 ± 3.4	2.9 (60%)	0.9	<.0001
Stuck in severe emotions related to the event	79	6.8 ± 2.5	2.6 ± 2.5	4.3 (63%)	1.7	<.0001
Suicidal thoughts	80	4.1 ± 3.3	0.9 ± 3.3	3.1 (77%)	1.0	<.0001
Aggregate score		7.0 ± 2.7	2.9 ± 2.7	4.1 (59%)	1.5	<.0001

SD: standard deviation.
* Bolded p-values indicate significance.

Improvement in PTSD related symptoms and pain

From baseline to follow-up, a highly significant reduction greater than the MCID was observed in the mean severity of all PTSD symptoms (p<0.0001) (Table 5). The aggregate score of PTSD symptoms were reduced from a mean score of 7.0 to 2.9 (59% reduction, ES 1.5, very large effect; p<0.0001). Notably, suicidal thoughts decreased from a baseline score of 4.1 to a follow-up score of 0.9 (77% reduction, ES 1.0, large effect; p<0.0001). Additionally, anxiety was reduced from a mean score of 7.8 to 3.3 (59% reduction, ES 9.0, very large effect; p<0.0001) and depression was reduced from 7.3 to 2.9 (60% reduction, ES 2.1, very large effect; p<0.0001). A 63% reduction in the mean score for anger and irritability was observed (7.9 to 3.0, ES 2.4, very large effect; p<0.0001). Pain severity decreased from an average of 6.6 (standard deviation (SD) 2.1) to 3.4 (SD 2.1) (48% reduction, ES 1.5, very large effect; n=80).

Impact of PTSD on social and family life

The severity of the impact of PTSD on social and family life was significantly reduced across all domains, with reductions in severity ranging from 46% to 82% (p≤0.0001) (Table 6). For all domains, improvement from baseline to follow-up was larger than the MCID. The aggregate score for the impact of PTSD on domains of social and family life decreased from 6.5 to 2.7 (59% reduction, ES 1.2, large effect; p<0.0001). Specifically, the mean score for the impact of PTSD on drug and alcohol overuse decreased from 6.0 to 1.1 (82% reduction, ES 1.4, very large effect; p<0.0001) and marital/relationship harmony was reduced from 8.1 to 2.8 (65% reduction, ES 2.6, very large effect; p<0.0001). A 48% reduction in the severity of the impact of PTSD on relationships with siblings and parents was also observed (7.1 to 3.7, ES 1.2, large effect; p<0.0001).

Table 6. Impact of PTSD on several domains of social and family life at baseline and follow-up (Scale of 0-10)

Impacted domain	Number of responses	Mean baseline score ± SD	Mean follow-up score ± SD	Improve-ment (%)	Effect size	p-value*
Drug and alcohol overuse	66	6.0 ± 3.6	1.1 ± 1.7	4.9 (82%)	1.4	<.0001
Marital or relationship harmony	70	8.1 ± 2.0	2.8 ± 2.4	5.3 (65%)	2.6	<.0001
Relationship with brothers / sisters / parents	73	7.1 ± 2.8	3.7 ± 2.6	3.4 (48%)	1.2	<.0001
Your belief that good things will happen in the future	72	6.1 ± 3.1	3.0 ± 2.3	3.1 (50%)	1.0	<.0001
Your belief that you are a valuable and appreciated member of society	47	6.1 ± 2.9	3.3 ± 2.5	2.8 (46%)	1.0	<.0001
Your belief that you belong in the "Human Race" or your concepts of society	35	5.8 ± 3.1	2.3 ± 2.0	3.4 (59%)	1.1	<.0001
Your relationship with children	66	6.7 ± 2.9	2.3 ± 2.3	4.3 (65%)	1.5	<.0001
Your trust in the relationship with "the creator" or your concept of "God"	51	5.7 ± 3.8	3.0 ± 2.9	2.8 (48%)	0.7	0.0001
Aggregate score		6.5 ± 3.1	2.7 ± 2.5	3.9 (59%)	1.2	<.0001

SD: Standard deviation.
* Bolded p-values indicate significance.

Table 7. Number of PTSD related medications at baseline and at follow-up, for patients with medication lists available (n=87)

Number of PTSD related medications	Number of patients on medications at baseline visit	Number of patients on medications at follow-up visit
0	28 (32%)	43 (49%)
1	11 (13%)	17 (20%)
2	13 (15%)	11 (13%)
3	12 (14%)	4 (5%)
4	13 (15%)	8 (9%)
5 or more	10 (11%)	4 (5%)

Reduction in PTSD related medication use

PTSD related medication information was available for 87 of 100 patients (Table 7). Of these 87 patients, 59 (68%) were using an average of 3.2 (SD 1.9) PTSD-related medications at baseline. At follow-up, the number of medications for these patients was reduced to an average of 1.6 (SD 1.8). The percentage of patients on two or more medications dropped from 55% at baseline to 31% at follow-up. Correspondingly, the percentage of patients on zero or one medication increased from 45% to 69% between baseline and follow-up. Of those 59 patients on PTSD-related medications at baseline, 21 (36%) had discontinued all PTSD related medications at follow-up, 19 (32%) had discontinued some of their PTSD medications, 14 (24%) had no change to their PTSD related medications, and 5 (8%) added some PTSD related medications.

DISCUSSION

PTSD is a debilitating disorder with a lifetime prevalence of 9.2% in Canada (3). This trauma- and stressor-related disorder is even more prevalent in military and police veterans as they may be exposed to many traumatic events during their service (6). However, traditional treatment options are not always effective in this population. Preliminary clinical research suggests that medical cannabis may be an effective alternative therapy for these patients. Therefore, the aim of the present study was to assess the clinical utility and efficacy of medical cannabis in Canadian military and police veterans with PTSD following initiation of cannabis use, by examining a variety of relevant patient outcomes through a retrospective chart review.

Patients in the study used multiple strains of cannabis containing varying amounts of cannabidiol (CBD) and delta-9-tetrahydrocannabinol (THC). Specifically, THC is the most common constituent of the Cannabis plant, and is most known for its psychoactive effects. Additionally, THC is used in a clinical setting for its analgesic and anti-nausea effects (23). In comparison, CBD is a non-psychotropic cannabinoid with anti-epileptic, anti-inflammatory, anti-emetic, and muscle relaxing properties. As a result, cannabis strains with differing CBD and THC ratios may offer a variety of medical benefits to patients.

These cannabinoids bind with CB-1 and CB-2 receptors that are a part of the mammalian endocannabinoid system. This system is involved in the regulation of mood, appetite, sleep, memory, and emotional state (24). Therefore, activation of CB-1 and CB-2receptors via cannabinoid binding produce the desired clinical effects associated with cannabis use, such as appetite stimulation, muscle relaxation, pain and anxiety reduction, and mood regulation (24). Furthermore, PTSD patients may have abnormalities in CB-1 receptors and low levels of the endogenous cannabinoid, anandamide (19). Therefore, stimulation of the CB-1 pathway through medical cannabis is a potential treatment option for reducing PTSD related symptoms.

A literature review conducted by Walsh et al. on the use of medical cannabis in the management of mental health found very few studies reporting the effects of cannabis on PTSD symptoms (20). A retrospective chart review by Greer et al. (25) examined changes in CAPS (Clinically Administered PTSD Scale) scores of 80 PTSD patients and observed a greater than 75% reduction in CAPS symptom scores in patients when they were using medical cannabis compared to when they were not using cannabis (25). However, patients included in this study were pre-screened for entry to the New Mexico Medical Cannabis Program having already used cannabis, therefore knowing that their PTSD symptoms were reduced with its use. Additionally, cannabis-withdrawal syndrome may have exacerbated their PTSD symptoms when they were not on cannabis, possibly contributing to their positive findings. Therefore, these results are not representative of the effects of cannabis in the general PTSD population (25). Fraser observed a 72% cessation of nightmares or reduction in nightmare severity after nabilone treatment in 47 PTSD patients with a 2-year history of PTSD-related nightmares who didn't respond to standard treatment previously (26). In an open pilot study by Roitman et al. (27), significant reductions in symptom severity were observed in the CAPS hyperarousal symptom cluster, sleep quality, and frequency and severity of nightmares after 10 Israeli PTSD patients were treated with oral Δ9-tetrahydrocannabinol (THC) as an add-on treatment (27). The present study also observed improvements in PTSD symptoms following medical cannabis use. In particular, a decrease in suicidal thinking post-initiation of medical cannabis was observed. Additionally, patients experienced significant improvements in social and family life through the reduction of their PTSD symptoms.

In the present study, a majority of patients reduced the number of PTSD-related medications used between baseline and follow-up, while 21 patients (24%) had discontinued all PTSD-medications at follow-up. Upon pharmacoeconomic evaluation, the estimated annual savings from these 21 patients discontinuing these prescription medications would range from $48,600 to $78,600 based on average daily dose for these medications, the price of generic versus brand name products, and assuming a dispensing fee of $10 per month. This translates into an average savings of $2,300 to $3,800 per year per patient. If medical cannabis can be used as an equally effective first line treatment option or replacement for other conventional pharmacotherapies, the health-care costs and financial burden associated with PTSD treatment can be significantly reduced.

Several limitations exist in the present study. First, this study was limited to a single centre under the supervision of a single physician, to which patients were only referred if they failed pharmacotherapy and psychotherapy. Thus, this sample may not be representative of all veterans with PTSD. Additionally, information regarding hospital admissions or adverse events while using medical cannabis was not available, preventing any determination of the risks or side effects associated with cannabis use. Since this was a retrospective chart review, some patients were missing data for certain outcomes, and dosages of PTSD related medications were not always specified. This study also did not use a validated tool for assessment of PTSD symptoms, nor was information regarding patients' history of cannabis use or duration of PTSD collected.

CONCLUSION

The results of a retrospective chart review presented in this study indicate that medical cannabis may be an effective treatment option for military and police veterans with PTSD, particularly those for whom conventional pharmacotherapy and psychotherapy was ineffective. Cannabis use resulted in improvements across all PTSD symptoms, social and family outcomes, and pain severity. Furthermore, these improvements were associated with a 50% reduction in the use of PTSD-related medications between baseline and follow-up, providing significant cost-savings to both the patient and greater health care system. In addition, less drug or alcohol overuse was observed following the initiation of medical cannabis use. Given the widespread use of medical cannabis among Canadian PTSD patients, it is essential that the safety, efficacy and clinical utility of medical cannabis be validated through thorough clinical investigations. Future studies should consider involving larger sample sizes and controls to determine the efficacy of medical cannabis in reducing PTSD-related symptoms, both as a first-line and alternative treatment option.

ACKNOWLEDGMENTS

We thank the generous support of Bratty Family Fund, Michael and Karyn Goldstein Cancer Research Fund, Joey and Mary Furfari Cancer Research Fund, Pulenzas Cancer Research Fund, Joseph and Silvana Melara Cancer Research Fund, and Ofelia Cancer Research Fund. This study was conducted in collaboration with MedReleaf.

REFERENCES

[1]   American Psychiatric Association. Trauma- and stressor-related disorders. In: Diagnostic and statistical manual of mental disorders, Fifth edition. Arlington, VA: American Psychiatric Association, 2013.

[2]   Rapaport MH, Clary C, Fayyad R, Endicott J. Quality-of-life impairment in depressive and anxiety disorders. Am J Psychiatry2005;162(6):1171–8.

[3]   Van Ameringen M, Mancini C, Patterson B, Boyle MH. Post-traumatic stress disorder in Canada. CNS Neurosci Ther 2008;14(3):171–81.

[4]   Stein MB, Walker JR, Forde DR. Gender differences in susceptibility to posttraumatic stress disorder. Behav Res Ther 2000;38(6):619–28.

[5]   Frise S, Steingart A, Sloan M, Cotterchio M, Kreiger N. Psychiatric disorders and use of mental health services by Ontario women. Can J Psychiatry 2002;47(9):849–56.

[6]   Zamorski MA, Boulos D. The impact of the military mission in Afghanistan on mental health in the Canadian Armed Forces: a summary of research findings. Eur J Psychotraumatol 2014;5:23822.

[7]   Steckler T, Risbrough V. Pharmacological treatment of PTSD – Established and new approaches. Neuropharmacology 2012;62(2):617–27.

[8]   Reist C, Kauffmann CD, Haier RJ, Sangdahl C, DeMet EM, Chicz-DeMet A, et al. A controlled trial of desipramine in 18 men with posttraumatic stress disorder. Am J Psychiatry 1989;146(4):513–6.

[9]   Marmar CR, Schoenfeld F, Weiss DS, Metzler T, Zatzick D, Wu R, et al. Open trial of fluvoxamine treatment for combat-related posttraumatic stress disorder. J Clin Psychiatry 1996;57(Suppl 8):66-72.

[10]   Hidalgo R, Hertzberg MA, Mellman T, Petty F, Tucker P, Weisler R, et al. Nefazodone in post-traumatic stress disorder: results from six open-label trials. Int Clin Psychopharmacol 1999;14(2):61–8.

[11]   Shestatzky M, Greenberg D, Lerer B. A controlled trial of phenelzine in posttraumatic stress disorder. Psychiatry Res 1988;24(2):149–55.

[12] Davidson J, Kudler H, Smith R, Mahorney SL, Lipper S, Hammett E, et al. Treatment of posttraumatic stress disorder with amitriptyline and placebo. Arch Gen Psychiatry 1990;47(3):259–66.

[13] Zisook S, Chentsova-Dutton YE, Smith-Vaniz A, Kline NA, Ellenor GL, Kodsi AB, et al. Nefazodone in patients with treatment-refractory posttraumatic stress disorder. J Clin Psychiatry2000;61(3):203–8.

[14] Hertzberg MA, Feldman ME, Beckham JC, Kudler HS, Davidson JR. Lack of efficacy for fluoxetine in PTSD: a placebo controlled trial in combat veterans. Ann Clin Psychiatry 2000;12(2):101–5.

[15] van der Kolk BA, Dreyfuss D, Michaels M, Shera D, Berkowitz R, Fisler R, et al. Fluoxetine in posttraumatic stress disorder. J Clin Psychiatry 1994;55(12):517–22.

[16] Zohar J, Amital D, Miodownik C, Kotler M, Bleich A, Lane RM, et al. Double-blind placebo-controlled pilot study of sertraline in military veterans with posttraumatic stress disorder. J Clin Psychopharmacol2002;22(2):190–5.

[17] Brady K, Pearlstein T, Asnis GM, Baker D, Rothbaum B, Sikes CR, et al. Efficacy and safety of sertraline treatment of posttraumatic stress disorder: a randomized controlled trial. JAMA 2000;283(14):1837–44.

[18] Davidson JR, Rothbaum BO, van der Kolk BA, Sikes CR, Farfel GM. Multicenter, double-blind comparison of sertraline and placebo in the treatment of posttraumatic stress disorder. Arch Gen Psychiatry 2001;58(5):485–92.

[19] Neumeister A, Normandin MD, Pietrzak RH, Piomelli D, Zheng MQ, Gujarro-Anton A, et al. Elevated brain cannabinoid CB1 receptor availability in post-traumatic stress disorder: a positron emission tomography study. Mol Psychiatry 2013;18(9):1034–40.

[20] Walsh Z, Gonzalez R, Crosby K, S. Thiessen M, Carroll C, Bonn-Miller MO. Medical cannabis and mental health: A guided systematic review. Clin Psychol Rev 2017;51:15–29.

[21] Cohen J. Statistical power analysis for the behavioral sciences, 2nd edition. Hillsdale, NJ: Lawrence Erlbaum,1988.

[22] Norman G, Sloan J, Wyrwich K. Interpretation of changes in health-related quality of life: the remarkable universality of half a standard deviation. Med Care 2003;41(5):582–92.

[23] Hazekamp A, Grotenhermen F. Review on clinical studies with cannabis and cannabinoids 2005-2009. Cannabinoids 2010;5(special issue):1–21.

[24] Grotenhermen F. The cannabinoid system-A brief review. J Ind Hemp 2004;9(2):87–92.

[25] Greer GR, Grob CS, Halberstadt AL. PTSD symptom reports of patients evaluated for the New Mexico Medical Cannabis Program. J Psychoactive Drugs2014;46(1):73–7.

[26] Fraser GA. The use of a synthetic cannabinoid in the management of treatment-resistant nightmares in Posttraumatic Stress Disorder (PTSD). CNS Neurosci Ther 2009;15(1):84–8.

[27] Roitman P, Mechoulam R, Cooper-Kazaz R, Shalev A. Preliminary, open-label, pilot study of add-on oral Δ9-tetrahydrocannabinol in chronic Post-Traumatic Stress Disorder. Clin Drug Investig 2014;34(8):587–91.

In: Medical Cannabis   ISBN: 978-1-53611-907-7
Editors: S. O'Hearn, A. Blake et al. © 2017 Nova Science Publishers, Inc.

Chapter 9

THE EFFECT OF MEDICAL CANNABIS ON ALCOHOL AND TOBACCO USE IN VETERANS WITH POST-TRAUMATIC STRESS DISORDER (PTSD)

Shicheng Jin[1], MD(C), Bo Angela Wan[1], MPhil,
Stephanie Chan[1], BSc(C), Paul A Smith[2], MD,
Alexia Blake[3], MSc, Amiti Wolt[3], BA,
Liying Zhang[1], PhD, Henry Lam[1], MLS,
Carlo DeAngelis[1], PharmD, Marissa Slaven[3], MD,
Erynn Shaw[3], MD, Vithusha Ganesh[1], BSc(C),
Pearl Zaki[1], BSc(C), Leah Drost[1], BSc(C),
Nicholas Lao[1], BMSc(C), Leila Malek[1], BSc(Hons),
Edward Chow[1], MBBS and Shannon O'Hearn[3],[*], MSc

---

[*] Correspondence: Ms Shannon O'Hearn MSc, MedReleaf Corp, Markham Industrial Park, Markham ON, Canada. Email: sohearn@medreleaf.com.

[1]Odette Cancer Centre, Sunnybrook Health Sciences Centre, University
of Toronto, Toronto, Ontario
[2]Dr Paul Smith Professional Corporation, Fredericton, New Brunswick
[3]MedReleaf, Markham, Ontario, Canada
[4]Juravinski Cancer Centre, Hamilton Health Sciences, Hamilton,
Ontario, Canada

Post-traumatic stress disorder (PTSD) is a mental illness that commonly
affects military and police service veterans after experiencing traumatic
events throughout their service. Alcohol and tobacco are often overused
by this population to help relieve the symptoms of PTSD. The objective
of this chapter is to examine if alcohol and tobacco use in military and
police service veterans with PTSD changed after using medical cannabis
for PTSD symptom management. A retrospective chart review was
conducted to analyse information about alcohol, tobacco, and medical
cannabis use, as well as previously attempted PTSD treatment methods.
101 patients (average age 43 years, 96.0% male, 60.4% married, and
81.2% with children) who visited a single treatment center between
January 2014 and April 2016 were included in this study. The most
common treatments patients tried prior to using medical cannabis
included self-treatment with non-medical cannabis (87.8%), medication
for depression (86.6%) and anxiety (85.4%), and psychotherapy (82.9%).
At baseline, 81.2% consumed alcohol (average 8.1 drinks/week) and
84.2% smoked tobacco cigarettes (average 2.7 packs/week). At follow-
up, 67.3% consumed alcohol (average 5.5 drinks/week) and 67.3%
smoked tobacco cigarettes (average 2.5 packs/week). The use of medical
cannabis was correlated with a reduction in alcohol and tobacco use.
However, statistical significance was not reached ($p=0.11$ and $p=0.65$,
respectively). Medical cannabis has the potential to reduce alcohol or
tobacco use in PTSD patients. Further investigation is required to
understand how medical cannabis can alleviate PTSD-related symptoms,
and to identify its impact on other lifestyle factors, such as tobacco and
alcohol consumption.

INTRODUCTION

Post-Traumatic Stress Disorder (PTSD), as defined by the "Diagnostic and
statistical manual of mental disorders, 5th edition" (DSM-V), is a

debilitating mental illness caused by experiencing or witnessing traumatic events such as sexual assault, violence, or personal grief. Symptoms of this condition include re-experiencing the pain and psychological stress of previous trauma, numbing or avoidance, and negative cognitions and mood (1).

Due to the nature of their lines of duty, military and police service veterans are more likely to experience PTSD than the general civilian population. In a literature review by Zamorski et al. of mental health within the Canadian Armed Forces, the prevalence of PTSD ranged from 2.1% to 8.1% in a study population of 8,400 personnel (2). Over a 4-year follow-up, 8% to 20% of Canadian Forces veterans were diagnosed with PTSD at some point during their service (2).

There is strong evidence suggesting that individuals with PTSD experience poorer health outcomes that reduce their quality of life (QOL) compared to individuals who do not have PTSD (3). For example, Rapaport et al. (4) reported that 59% of PTSD patients have clinically significant severe impairments in QOL items compared to non-PTSD populations, as defined by two or more standard deviations below the community norm. QOL reductions in PTSD populations are even more severe than patients with panic disorder, obsessive compulsive disorder, and social phobia (4). In military and police veterans with PTSD, a deterioration in QOL, in combination with chronic symptoms of PTSD can lead to social or occupational impairment, resulting in an inability to successfully resume a civilian lifestyle (4).

Population studies in the United States have revealed associations between nicotine and alcohol dependence in individuals with psychiatric disorders (5). According to the DSM-V guidelines, nicotine or alcohol dependence is defined as the presence of at least 2 out of 11 criteria that evaluate characteristics of nicotine or alcohol intake (1). Breslau et al. (6) reported that in persons with PTSD, there is an increased risk of nicotine dependence, as PTSD patients may find that nicotine helps them cope with PTSD-related symptoms (6). Despite anecdotal evidence suggesting that alcohol is often used to cope with their symptoms as well, there is mixed evidence regarding the risk of alcohol abuse or dependence in individuals with PTSD (6, 7).

Conventionally, PTSD is treated and managed with pharmacotherapy and psychotherapy. Common pharmacotherapies include tricyclic antidepressants, adrenoceptor agonists or antagonists, anticonvulsants, antipsychotics, selective serotonin reuptake inhibitors (SSRIs), and monoamine oxidase inhibitors (7). However, traditional pharmacotherapy is inconsistently effective for treating combat-related PTSD compared to civilian PTSD, possibly due to the chronic nature of combat-related PTSD. In comparison, psychotherapy may be a more a consistently effective treatment option for patients with all types of PTSD, often resulting in significant symptom improvements (3, 8–14). Meta-analyses of 26 studies of the efficacy of psychotherapy treatments ranging from 3-52 hours in length suggested that over 67% of PTSD patients no longer met the criteria for PTSD after treatment completion (9).

Recently, medical cannabis has emerged as an effective alternative treatment option for patients suffering from PTSD, particularly among the military veteran population. While its efficacy is beginning to be formally investigated in this population, the current literature lacks evidence supporting whether the use of medical cannabis specifically reduces alcohol and tobacco use in military and policy veterans with PTSD. The objective of this chapter was to address this gap in the literature to understand whether the use of medical cannabis is correlated with a reduction in alcohol and tobacco use in Canadian military and police veterans with PTSD.

OUR RESEARCH

A retrospective chart audit was conducted at a single medical practice in New Brunswick, Canada, with experience in managing PTSD in military veterans. The charts of 101 patients who had begun treatment with medical cannabis between January 2014 and January 2016 were assessed in this study. These patients had a confirmed diagnosis of PTSD, served in the military or police service, and had failed previous attempts of pharmacotherapy and psychotherapy. Patients were started on a medical cannabis dose of 1 gram/day, and self-titrated until desired results were met. Daily doses did not exceed 10 grams/day.

Patient charts were retrospectively reviewed to analyze information recorded at baseline (initial visit) and at first follow-up. At baseline, demographic information including age, gender, marital status, number of children, length of military or police service, family history of medical conditions, and past medical histories were recorded. In addition, medications (type and dose), and weekly alcohol and tobacco use were documented. Patients were also asked to describe their history of PTSD, whether they experienced pain as a symptom, the location of pain on their body, and to rate the efficacy of previous treatments for PTSD symptoms on a scale of 1 to 10, with 10 being most effective. Previous treatments that were rated included psychotherapy, relaxation therapy, exercise programs, nutrition therapy, medications for anxiety, medications for depression, self-treatment with non-medical cannabis, and isolation to a place in nature.

At follow-up, information including time to follow-up, current medications (type and dose), previous treatment efficacy, presence of pain, and location of pain were documented. Details of medical cannabis use including the duration of cannabis use, median daily dose, method of cannabis administration (smoking, vaping, or eating), and cannabis strain(s) used were recorded. Finally, alcohol consumption and tobacco consumption per week were reported.

Changes in the average score and significance for outcome across all participants from baseline to the first follow-up were analyzed. For each outcome, any patient responses in the form of a numerical range (ex. "6-8 out of 10 for shoulder pain") were represented by the median. A two-tailed unpaired t-test was used to analyze alcohol and tobacco use between baseline and follow-up, with significance defined as $p<0.05$.

WHAT WE FOUND

Table 1 shows baseline demographic data of the 101 patients assessed. Patients were primarily male (96.0%) and on average 43 years old. Over sixty percent were married, 14.9% were in a common-law relationship, 11.9% were either divorced/separated or single, and the relationship status of 1.0% was unknown. Of the 81.2% of patients who had children, the average number of children per patient was 2.2.

Table 1. Baseline information on patient demographics

Demographics (Total n=101)	n (%)
Average age (years)	43 (SD=9.8)
Sex (Total n=101)	97 Male (96.0%)
Marital status	
Married	61 (60.4%)
Common law	15 (14.9%)
Divorced/separated	12 (11.9%)
Single	12 (11.9%)
Unknown	1 (1.0%)
Children	
Number of patients with children	82 (81.2%)
Average number of children	2.2 (SD=1.0)
Military service	
Average length of military/police service (years)	16.2 (SD=7.8)
Common family history of medical illness	
Diabetes	33 (32.7%)
Cancer	30 (29.7%)
Heart disease	20 (49.5%)
Depression	12 (11.9%)
High blood pressure	7 (6.9%)
Post-traumatic stress disorder	6 (5.9%)
Common locations of pain (Total n=89)	
Back	50 (62.1%)
Shoulder	28 (31.5%)
Knee	28 (31.5%)
Neck	20 (22.5%)
Ankle	11 (12.4%)

SD: standard deviation.

The effect of medical cannabis on alcohol and tobacco use ...   139

The average length of military and police service of patients involved in this study was 16.2 years. Patients most commonly had a family history of diabetes (32.7%), cancer (29.7%), heart disease (19.8%), depression (11.9%), high blood pressure (6.9%), and PTSD (5.9%).

Table 2. Prevalence and effectiveness of previous PTSD treatments (Total n=82)

Treatment	n (%)	Average score (0-10)	SD
Self-treatments with non-medical cannabis on your own	72 (87.8%)	8.53	2.34
Medication for depression	71 (86.6%)	3.99	2.68
Medication for anxiety	70 (85.4%)	4.24	2.81
Psychotherapy	68 (82.9%)	5.15	2.66
No treatment	57 (69.5%)	2.94	2.91
Isolation to a place in nature	55 (67.1%)	6.64	3.26
Exercise programs of any sort	52 (63.4%)	5.00	2.79
Relaxation therapy (ex. Meditation, Yoga)	42 (51.2%)	4.26	2.94
Nutrition therapy	20 (24.4%)	1.90	2.72

SD: Standard deviation.

Table 1 shows that out of the 89 patients experiencing pain at baseline, most patients reported experiencing pain in their back (62.1%), shoulder (31.5%), knee (31.5%), neck (22.5%), and ankle (12.4%). The average time to follow-up with patients was 8.25 months (SD=4.9).

Previous treatment prevalence and effectiveness

Previous treatments are listed in Table 2, and include self-treatment with non-medical cannabis (87.8%), medication for depression (86.6%), medication for anxiety (85.4%), psychotherapy (82.9%), no treatment (69.5%), isolation to a place in nature (67.1%), exercise programs (63.4%), relaxation therapy (51.2%), and nutrition therapy (24.4%). The self-perceived efficacies of these treatments ranged widely. The three most effective treatment methods include self-treatment with non-medical cannabis (efficacy score=8.5), isolation to a place in nature (efficacy score=6.6), and psychotherapy (efficacy score=5.2).

Table 3. Preferred method of medical cannabis use (Total n=97)

Method of use	n (%)
Vaporize	80 (82.5%)
Smoke	77 (79.4%)
Oral consumption	63 (64.9%)

Medical cannabis use

The median daily dose patients reported to be using at follow-up was 10 grams/day. Table 3 shows that the preferred methods of administration included vaporization (82.5%), smoking (79.4%), and ingestion (64.9%). The top five varieties of cannabis supplied from *MedReleaf Corp.* that patients perceived provided the greatest relief overall include *Luminarium*^{MR} (36.0%), *Sedamen*^{MR} (32.6%), *Avidekel*^{MR} (27.9%), *Midnight*^{MR} (26.7%), and *Remissio*^{MR}(24.4%) (see Table 4).

Table 4. Top 5 preferred varieties of medical cannabis by patients and characteristics (Total n=86)

Variety	n (%)	Composition	% THC	% CBD	$/gram
Luminarium^{MR}	31 (36.0%)	Very *sativa-*dominant	25 - 28%	0	12.5
Sedamen^{MR}	28 (32.6%)	*indica*-dominant	21 - 24%	0	12.5
Avidekel^{MR}	24 (27.9%)	*sativa*-leaning	8 - 11%	11 - 14%	12.5
Midnight^{MR}	23 (26.7%)	*indica*-leaning	0.1 - 0.8%	15 - 18%	12.5
Remissio^{MR}	21 (24.4%)	*indica*-dominant	24 - 27%	0	12.5

THC: Tetrahydrocannabinol; CBD: cannabidiol.

Table 5. Average alcohol and tobacco use at baseline and follow-up

Alcohol use (drinks/week)		
Baseline (n=81)	Follow-up (n=81)	p-value
8.1 (SD=10.7)	5.5 (SD=9.5)	0.11
Tobacco use (packs/week)		
Baseline (n=68)	Follow-up (n=68)	p-value
2.7 (SD=2.9)	2.5 (SD=3.1)	0.65

SD: standard deviation.

Improvement in alcohol and tobacco use

At baseline, patients reported consuming and average of 8.1 drinks/week, compared to 5.5 drinks/week at follow-up (p=0.11, Table 5). Patients consumed an average of 2.7 packs of cigarettes/week at baseline, compared to 2.5 packs/week at follow-up (p=0.65). Neither of these changes reached statistical significance.

DISCUSSION

PTSD is a debilitating disorder caused by witnessing or experiencing a traumatic event, and has a lifetime prevalence of 9.2% in Canada (10). PTSD is more prevalent in military and police veteran populations since they are more likely to be exposed to traumatic events during their service in comparison to the civilian population (10). PTSD may manifest as a variety of symptoms such as depression and pain, as well as dependence on substances such as alcohol and tobacco. These have long-term psychosocial consequences as well as a negative impact on QOL (5, 12, 13).

PTSD patients may be at an increased risk of nicotine and alcohol dependence, as defined by the DSM-5. Breslau et al. reported that an increased prevalence of nicotine dependence observed in PTSD patients may be due to the ability of nicotine to help patients cope with their PTSD symptoms of re-experiencing trauma and hyper-arousal (6, 7, 13). Nicotine dependence is linked to an increased risk of short-term and long-term health outcomes through affecting the respiratory and gastrointestinal systems, as well as cognition (5, 15, 16).

Twin studies have identified PTSD as a significant risk factor for alcohol dependence, possibly due to its ability to help patients cope with PTSD symptoms such as insomnia (6, 16). Alcohol dependence adversely impacts health through negatively affecting cognition and causing liver damage (17). As PTSD patients may be more prone to alcohol and tobacco dependence, there is a higher risk that this patient group will encounter additional health problems, which may further impact their QOL and general wellbeing (14). Moreover, Cocker et al. (24) found that among veterans with PTSD, there was a correlation between a three-way reduction of PTSD symptoms, substance abuse issues, and violent behaviour, suggesting a synergistic mechanism underlying these issues (24). Therefore, management of PTSD symptoms as well as reduction of substance dependence is critical for improving the overall health of these patients.

Medical cannabis is emerging as an effective alternative treatment option for the management of a wide variety of symptoms, including those associated with PTSD. The results presented in this study suggest that the use of medical cannabis may also lead to a reduction in tobacco and alcohol use in veteran PTSD patient populations. It is important to further investigate the short and long-term effects of medical cannabis on alcohol, tobacco, and possibly other substance abuse, especially since PTSD patients may display a higher tendency to develop alcohol and tobacco dependency (12). While the present study provides valuable insight into the potential of medical cannabis to reduce alcohol and tobacco use in military and police veterans experiencing PTSD, further research is required to understand the complete effects of medical cannabis on symptom management and substance abuse mitigation in both PTSD and non-PTSD populations.

The literature portrays mixed evidence regarding the efficacy of traditional treatment methods such as psychotherapy and pharmacotherapy for managing PTSD-associated symptoms (9, 18, 19). Similarly, patients in this study reported varying efficacies of other forms of treatment, many of which had limited success and therefore led patients to seek further treatment at this center (see Table 2). However, since patients included in this study were military and police veterans, the results of this study may not be directly applicable to non-veteran subgroups of the PTSD patient population.

Several limitations apply to this present study. First, this study was limited to a single center under the supervision of a single physician. As patients were only referred to this center if they failed pharmacotherapy and psychotherapy, this sample population displaying treatment resistance may not be representative of all veterans or civilians with PTSD. Additionally, some patients had missing or incomplete data for certain outcomes and dosages of PTSD-related medications, which may also have affected study observations. Outcomes were also recorded by the physician based on consultation with the patient, and objective validated tools were not used, potentially introducing biases into the data. In the future, larger study cohorts, consistent follow-up intervals, and the use of objective tools to collect symptom and QOL related measures will help further the understanding of whether the use of medical cannabis has significant impacts on alcohol and tobacco use patients with PTSD.

CONCLUSION

The results from this retrospective chart review provide early findings that cannabis may be an effective treatment option for military and police veterans with PTSD, especially those who did not respond to other conventional therapies. Although statistical significance was not observed, medical cannabis use in this cohort was correlated with a reduction in alcohol and tobacco use. Further research is required with larger populations and study controls to determine the efficacy of medical cannabis in managing PTSD-related symptoms and as a long-term method for mitigating substance abuse in both PTSD and non-PTSD patient populations.

ACKNOWLEDGMENTS

We thank the generous support of Bratty Family Fund, Michael and Karyn Goldstein Cancer Research Fund, Joey and Mary Furfari Cancer Research Fund, Pulenzas Cancer Research Fund, Joseph and Silvana Melara Cancer Research Fund, and Ofelia Cancer Research Fund. This study was conducted in collaboration with MedReleaf.

REFERENCES

[1] American Psychiatric Association. Trauma- and stressor-related disorders. In: Diagnostic and Statistical Manual of Mental Disorders, Fifth edition. Arlington, VA: American Psychiatric Association, 2013.

[2] Zamorski MA, Boulos D. The impact of the military mission in afghanistan on mental health in the Canadian Armed Forces: A summary of research findings. Eur J Psychotraumatol 2014;5.

[3] Mendlowicz M V, Stein MB. Reviews and Overviews Quality of Life in Individuals With Anxiety Disorders. Psychiatry Interpers Biol Process 2000;157(5):669–82.

[4] Rapaport MH, Clary C, Fayyad R, Endicott J. Quality-of-Life Impairment in Depressive and Anxiety Disorders. Am J Psychiatry 2005;162(6):1171–8.

[5] Grant BF, Hasin DS, Chou SP, Stinson FS, Dawson DA. Nicotine dependence and psychiatric disorders in the United States. Arch Gen Psychiatry 2004;61(11):1107-15.

[6] Breslau N, Davis GC, Schultz LR. Posttraumatic stress disorder and the incidence of nicotine, alcohol, and other drug disorders in persons who have experienced trauma. Arch Gen Psychiatry 2003;60(3):289–94.

[7] Veteran Administration. PTSD and substance abuse in veterans, 2014. URL: http://www.ptsd.va.gov/public/problems/ptsd_substance_abuse_veterans.asp.

[8] Steckler T, Risbrough V. Pharmacological treatment of PTSD: Established and new approaches. Neuropharmacol 2012;62(2):617–27.

[9] Bradley R, Ph D, Greene J, Russ E, Dutra L, Westen D, et al. Reviews and Overviews A Multidimensional Meta-Analysis of Psychotherapy for PTSD. Am J Psychiatry 2005;162:214–27.

[10] Van Ameringen M, Mancini C, Patterson B, Boyle MH. Post-traumatic stress disorder in Canada. CNS Neurosci Ther 2008;14(3):171–81.

[11] Walsh Z, Callaway R, Belle-Isle L, Capler R, Kay R, Lucas P, et al. Cannabis for therapeutic purposes: Patient characteristics, access, and reasons for use. Int J Drug Policy 2013;24(6):511–6.

[12] Feldner MT, Babson KA, Zvolensky MJ. Critical Review of the Empirical Literature. October 2008;27(1):14–45.

[13] Stewart SH, Mitchell TL, Wright KD, Loba P. The relations of PTSD symptoms to alcohol use and coping drinking in volunteers who responded to the Swissair Flight 111 airline disaster. J Anxiety Disord 2004;18(1):51–68.

[14] McFarlane AC. Epidemiological evidence about the relationship between PTSD and alcohol abuse: The nature of the association. Addict Behav 1998;23(6):813–25.

[15] Babson KA, Feldner MT, Sachs-Ericsson N, Schmidt NB, Zvolensky MJ. Nicotine dependence mediates the relations between insomnia and both panic and posttraumatic stress disorder in the NCS-R sample. Depress Anxiety 2008;25 (8):670–9.

[16] Koenen KC, Hitsman B, Lyons MJ, Niaura R, McCaffery J, Goldberg J, et al. A twin registry study of the relationship between posttraumatic stress disorder and nicotine dependence in men. Arch Gen Psychiatry 2005;62(11):1258–65.

[17] World Health Organization. Alcohol. Geneva: WHO, 2015. URL: http://www.who.int/mediacentre/factsheets/fs349/en/%0Afiles/372/en.html.

[18] Hetrick SE, Purcell R, Garner B, Parslow R. Combined pharmacotherapy and psychological therapies for post traumatic stress disorder (PTSD). CochraneDatabaseSystRev 2010;7:CD007316.

[19] Foa E, Meaows EA. Psychosocial treatments for posttraumatic stress disorder: A critical review. Annu Rev Psychol 1997;48:449–80.

In: Medical Cannabis   ISBN: 978-1-53611-907-7
Editors: S. O'Hearn, A. Blake et al.   © 2017 Nova Science Publishers, Inc.

Chapter 10

THE EFFICACY OF DIFFERENT VARIETIES OF MEDICAL CANNABIS IN RELIEVING SYMPTOMS IN POST-TRAUMATIC STRESS DISORDER (PTSD) PATIENTS

Leah Drost[1], BSc(C), Bo Angela Wan[1], MPhil,
Alexia Blake[2], MSc, Stephanie Chan[1], BSc(C),
Amiti Wolt[2], BA, Vithusha Ganesh[1], BSc(C),
Liying Zhang[1], PhD, Marissa Slaven[3], MD,
Erynn Shaw[3], MD, Carlo DeAngelis[1], PharmD,
Henry Lam[1], MLS, Pearl Zaki[1], BSc(C),
Leila Malek[1], BSc(Hons), Edward Chow[1], MBBS
and Shannon O'Hearn[2,*], MSc

[1]Odette Cancer Centre, Sunnybrook Health Sciences Centre,
University of Toronto, Toronto, Ontario
[2]MedReleaf, Markham, Ontario
[3]Juravinski Cancer Centre, Hamilton Health Sciences, Hamilton,
Ontario, Canada

---

* Correspondence: Ms. Shannon O'Hearn MSc, Project Manager, Clinical Research, MedReleaf, Markham Industrial Park, Markham, Ontario, Canada. Email: sohearn@medreleaf.com.

Post-traumatic stress disorder (PTSD) is a crippling condition that affects individuals who have experienced severe traumatic event(s). Cannabis is emerging as a treatment option for patients experiencing PTSD. The objective of this chapter is to determine which varieties of cannabis PTSD patients perceive to be most effective for relieving their symptoms. PTSD patients using medical cannabis from a Canadian licensed provider voluntarily completed an online survey at baseline, 4 and 10 months, which collected information pertaining to their medical conditions, symptoms, and use of medical cannabis. The majority of PTSD patients reported improvement in all most commonly reported symptoms, including depression, anxiety, sleep problems, and pain, following the use of medical cannabis (p<0.0001). *Sedamen*^{MR} was reported to be effective in relieving overall PTSD at 4 and 10 months, and also helped manage each of the four common symptoms. *Luminarium*^{MR} was also reported to be beneficial for PTSD at 4 and 10 months, as well as for depression, anxiety, and pain. *Alaska*^{MR} was reported beneficial for PTSD after 4 months as well as for depression, anxiety, and sleep problems. *Midnight*^{MR} was reported to be effective in relieving PTSD after 10 months, and also was reportedly beneficial for all four common symptoms. Study results demonstrated that PTSD patients perceived notable differences in the effectiveness of cannabis varieties for managing their symptoms. Further research in a controlled clinical setting to determine which varieties manage PTSD symptoms most effectively will help clinicians make better recommendations to patients.

INTRODUCTION

Post-traumatic stress disorder (PTSD) is a debilitating mental health condition with several manifestations that occurs in some people after experiencing a traumatic event. Predisposing factors have been identified, as not all individuals who are exposed to trauma will develop this condition (1). Several different types of psychotherapy and pharmacotherapy treatment options are available for PTSD and its associated symptoms such as hyperarousal, re-experiencing traumatic events, and avoidance (2, 3). The multifaceted physiology of PTSD must be taken into consideration when developing treatment plans.

The PTSD brain presents with modified circuitry and structural changes (1, 4, 5). Patients with PTSD also experience altered endocrine and neurochemical activity compared to non-PTSD patients. The neurochemical changes in PTSD patients often manifest as a dysregulation of several neurotransmitters including catecholamines and serotonin. As neurochemical regulation plays an important role in a wide range of brain functions, including the ability to form memories and process emotion, neurochemical imbalances can disturb the emotional control of PTSD patients.

Major dysregulation of the endocrine system also occurs in PTSD patients, specifically dysregulation of the glucocorticoid and thyroid hormone systems. The hypothalamic-pituitary-adrenal (HPA) axis is the body's stress regulation system. Each part of the axis works together to modulate the stress response through the release of a cascade of various hormones and ultimately, the release of glucocorticoids, including the body's main stress hormone, cortisol (1, 6). In a healthy brain, a negative feedback system regulates cortisol release to suppress the stress response after a stressful stimulus is no longer present. Studies have shown that PTSD patients have an increased negative feedback response however, leading to the release of lower levels of cortisol during periods of stress (1, 7). In addition, low cortisol levels before exposure to a traumatic event may predispose a person to developing PTSD (1, 8, 9). Some studies have also indicated that abnormal levels of thyroid hormones in PTSD patients can be associated with increased anxiety (1, 10).

Medical cannabis is emerging as a viable treatment option for patients with PTSD, as an alternative to, or in conjunction with, traditional psychotherapy and pharmacotherapy. Many different strains of medical cannabis exist, each with unique profiles of active compounds, namely cannabinoids. The two most well studied cannabinoids thought to be predominantly responsible for the physiologic effects of cannabis are tetrahydrocannabinol (THC) and cannabidiol (CBD). THC is the main psychoactive constituent, whereas CBD is non-psychoactive and thought to possess antipsychotic, anti-inflammatory, and anxiolytic properties (3, 11).

Medical cannabis varieties are derived from two main subspecies of cannabis - *Cannabis sativa* and *Cannabis indica*. In general, anecdotal evidence suggests that *sativa* dominant strains produce a more stimulating effect, whereas *indica* dominant varieties tend to be more sedative in nature (3). Varieties available to medical patients contain unique cannabinoid and *indica/sativa* properties, as well as profiles of other potentially physiologically active, but less well studied compounds such as terpenes. These different characteristics are likely to contribute to variations in the efficacy of strains for the management of various symptoms. As patients have access to such an array of cannabis strains, it is important to establish which are most effective for PTSD symptom management from a clinical perspective. The varieties of medical cannabis in this study were classified per their relative composition of *indica* and *sativa*. For example, varieties were categorized as *sativa*-leaning (consisting of 50-60% *sativa*), *sativa*-dominant (61-70% *sativa*), or very *sativa*-dominant (>70% *sativa*); *indica* varieties were categorized similarly.

OUR STUDY

Patients registered with a Canadian licensed cannabis provider were invited to complete a voluntary online survey upon registration with the provider (baseline), and at 4- and 10-month follow-up intervals.

The online survey was developed by a licensed cannabis producer in consultation with various healthcare professionals with knowledge of medical cannabis, for the purpose of gathering information about patient demographics, quality of life, current symptoms and conditions, and the use and preference of different medical cannabis varieties. Surveys were dynamic, and follow-up questions were customized based on answers to previous questions. Patients were able to skip questions, and could select more than one answer for several questions. As a result, each patient answered a unique set of questions. The average completion time was between 15-25 minutes.

Patients were invited to complete an intake survey at the time of registration with the licensed provider (baseline). Questions were designed to collect information pertaining to demographics, current conditions and symptoms, and corresponding severities. Patients were also asked to report on their quality of life, which related to their experience with a number of key activities of daily living (ADLs).

At 4 and 10 months from baseline, patients were invited to complete follow-up surveys, in which they were asked questions about any changes to their symptoms or conditions, their experience with cannabis treatment, and which varieties they perceived to have had the greatest effect. There were no restrictions on the number of varieties each respondent could select.

All surveys included in this analysis were completed between January 2015 and December 2016. 3,076 patients in total completed the survey at baseline, of which 647 patients reported having PTSD.

Descriptive and inferential statistical analyses were performed. Along with basic statistics such as mean and range calculations, the Fisher exact test was performed to determine significance of symptom improvement and volume of usage of medical cannabis when comparing PTSD with non-PTSD patients. A p-value of less than 0.05 was considered statistically significant.

FINDINGS

3,076 patients completed baseline surveys, 647 of which reported experiencing PTSD. At baseline, the four most commonly reported symptoms for all patients including those with PTSD were pain (74.3%), anxiety (74.0%), sleep problems (71.4%), and depression (60.4%).

Perceived changes in the condition (PTSD) and commonly experienced symptoms following medical cannabis use are shown in Table 1. Of 171 patients with PTSD reporting a change in their condition following the use of cannabis, 12.3% responded that their condition deteriorated between baseline and 4-month follow-up. 10.5% of PTSD patients reported no change in their condition, while the remaining 77.2% indicated that their condition had improved following the use of cannabis (p=0.0031).

Table 1. Change in severity of PTSD and the four most commonly experienced symptoms of PTSD patients

	Deterioration, n (%)	No change, n (%)	Improvement, n (%)	No longer experiencing this symptom, n (%)	p-value*
PTSD (Total n=171)	21 (12.3%)	18 (10.5%)	132 (77.2%)	N/A	**0.0031**
Depression (Total n=143)	16 (11.2%)	15 (10.5%)	111 (77.6%)	1 (0.7%)	**<0.0001**
Anxiety (Total n=157)	18 (11.5%)	15 (9.6%)	123 (78.3%)	1 (0.6%)	**<0.0001**
Sleep problems (Total n=142)	16 (11.3%)	20 (14.1%)	100 (70.4%)	6 (4.2%)	**<0.0001**
Pain (Total n=124)	10 (8.1%)	12 (9.7%)	100 (80.6%)	2 (1.6%)	**<0.0001**

PTSD – post traumatic stress disorder.
* Bolded p-values are statistically significant.

143 PTSD patients experiencing depression reported a change at the 4-month follow-up. 11.2% indicated that this symptom had deteriorated after using cannabis, 10.5% reported no change, and 77.6% responded that they had experienced improvement in their depression following the use of cannabis (p<0.0001). Additionally, 0.7% indicated that they no longer experienced this symptom. Of respondents experiencing anxiety (n=157), 11.5% indicated that their symptom deteriorated, 9.6% reported no change, 78.3% reported improvement, and 0.6% responded that they no longer experienced anxiety after 4 months (p<0.0001). 142 patients reported experiencing a change in their sleep problems at follow-up. 11.3% experienced a deterioration of this symptom, 14.1% reported no change, 70.4% reported experiencing an improvement, and 4.2% no longer experienced sleep problems (p<0.0001). Finally, 124 patients indicated experiencing a change in their pain following cannabis use. Of these patients, only 8.1% reported deterioration, and 9.7% reported experiencing no change in their pain levels. 80.6% of patients previously experiencing

pain indicated that their symptom had improved, and 1.6% reported no longer experiencing pain after using cannabis (p<0.0001).

PREFERRED VARIETIES FOR RELIEF OF PTSD

At the 4-month follow-up, 38 patients with PTSD indicated which varieties of cannabis they felt were most effective for their overall condition. 35 of these patients also provided responses at the 10-month follow-up. At 4-month follow-up, 39.5% of these respondents preferred *Stellio*[MR] (very *indica*-dominant, 23-26% THC, 0% CBD), while 31.6% indicated that *Sedamen*[MR] (very *indica*-dominant, 21-24% THC, 0% CBD), *Alaska*[MR] (very *sativa*-dominant, 20-23% THC, 0% CBD), and *Luminarium*[MR] (very *sativa*-dominant, 25-28% THC, 0% CBD) were most beneficial for managing their PTSD (Table 2).

At the 10-month follow-up, responses differed slightly. 48.6% of PTSD patients reported *Sedamen*[MR] to be most effective, 45.7% chose *Luminarium*[MR], 42.9% chose *Midnight*[MR] (*sativa*-leaning, 8-11% THC, 11-14% CBD), and 34.3% chose *Avidekel*[MR] (*indica*-leading, 0.1-0.8%, THC, 15-18% CBD). The compositions of *indica* and *sativa* species in each variety, as well as the levels of THC and CBD, are included in Table 2.

PREFERRED VARIETIES FOR RELIEF OF
COMMON PTSD SYMPTOMS

The most common symptoms experienced by all respondents at baseline, including PTSD patients, were depression, anxiety, sleep problems, and pain. Reported strain efficacy for each of these symptoms is shown in Table 3.

Table 2. Varieties most helpful for PTSD at 4 months and 10 months and composition of each variety (% *indica, sativa,* **THC, CBD)**

Variety	Number of patients who reported variety to be helpful n (%)	Composition	% THC	% CBD
4 months (Total n=38)				
Stellio[MR]	15 (39.5%)	very *indica*-dominant	23 - 26%	0
Sedamen[MR]	12 (31.6%)	very *indica*-dominant	21 - 24%	0
Alaska[MR]	12 (31.6%)	very *sativa*-dominant	20 - 23%	0
Luminarium[MR]	12 (31.6%)	very *sativa*-dominant	25 - 28%	0
10 months (Total n=35)				
Sedamen[MR]	17 (48.6%)	very *indica*-dominant	21 - 24%	0
Luminarium[MR]	16 (45.7%)	very *sativa*-dominant	25 - 28%	0
Midnight[MR]	15 (42.9%)	*sativa*-leaning	8 - 11%	11 - 14%
Avidekel[MR]	12 (34.3%)	*indica*-leaning	0.1 - 0.8%	15 - 18%

PTSD: post traumatic stress disorder; THC: tetrahydrocannabinol; CBD: cannabidiol.

Of 93 PTSD patients experiencing depression at the 4-month follow-up, 39.8% reported *Luminarium*[MR] to be most effective, 22.6% selected *Midnight*[MR] and *Sedamen*[MR], and 21.5% indicated *Alaska*[MR], *Voluptas*[MR] (very *sativa*-dominant, 20-23% THC, 0% CBD), and *Elevare*[MR] (very *sativa* dominant, 24-27% THC, 0% CBD) to be most effective in relieving this symptom. At 4 months from baseline, there were 110 patients with PTSD who indicated that they experienced anxiety. These patients reported that *Sedamen*[MR] (30.0%), *Luminarium*[MR] (29.1%), *Midnight*[MR] (26.4%), and *Alaska*[MR] (25.5%) were most effective in relieving this symptom. The third most common symptom experienced by PTSD patients was sleep problems (n = 89). Patients who reported experiencing problems with sleep indicated that *Sedamen*[MR] (34.8%), *Midnight*[MR] (23.6%), *Remissio*[MR] (very*indica*-dominant, 24-27% THC, 0% CBD; 23.6%), and *Alaska*[MR] (18.0%) were most effective in relieving this symptom. Finally, PTSD patients experiencing pain (n = 91) indicated that *Sedamen*[MR] (36.3%) was most beneficial in alleviating this symptom, followed by *Midnight*^(MR) (34.1%), *Luminarium*^(MR) (29.7%) and *Avidekel*^(MR) (29.7%).

Table 3. Varieties most helpful for PTSD symptoms and composition of each variety

Variety	Number of patients who reported variety to be helpful, n (%)	Composition	% THC	% CBD
Depression (Total n=93)				
Luminarium^(MR)	37 (39.8%)	very *sativa*-dominant	25 - 28%	0
Midnight^(MR)	21 (22.6%)	*sativa*-leaning	8 - 11%	11 - 14%
Sedamen^(MR)	21 (22.6%)	very *indica*-dominant	21 - 24%	0
Alaska^(MR)	20 (21.5%)	very *sativa*-dominant	20 - 23%	0
Voluptas^(MR)	20 (21.5%)	very *sativa*-dominant	20 - 23%	0
Elevare^(MR)	20 (21.5%)	very *sativa*-dominant	24 - 27%	0
Anxiety (Total n=110)				
Sedamen^(MR)	33 (30.0%)	very *indica*-dominant	21 - 24%	0
Luminarium^(MR)	32 (29.1%)	very *sativa*-dominant	25 - 28%	0
Midnight^(MR)	29 (26.4%)	*sativa*-leaning	8 - 11%	11 - 14%
Alaska^(MR)	28 (25.5%)	very *sativa*-dominant	20 - 23%	0
Sleep problems (Total n=89)				
Sedamen^(MR)	31 (34.8%)	very *indica*-dominant	21 - 24%	0
Midnight^(MR)	21 (23.6%)	*sativa*-leaning	8 - 11%	11 - 14%
Remissio^(MR)	21 (23.6%)	very *indica*-dominant	24 - 27%	0
Alaska^(MR)	16 (18.0%)	very *sativa*-dominant	20 - 23%	0
Pain (Total n=91)				
Sedamen^(MR)	33 (36.3%)	very *indica*-dominant	21 - 24%	0
Midnight^(MR)	31 (34.1%)	*sativa*-leaning	8 - 11%	11 - 14%
Luminarium^(MR)	27 (29.7%)	very *sativa*-dominant	25 - 28%	0
Avidekel^(MR)	27 (29.7%)	*indica*-leaning	0.1 - 0.8%	15 - 18%

THC: tetrahydrocannabinol; CBD: cannabidiol.

Table 4. Dosage of medical cannabis in PTSD versus non-PTSD patients

Dose	Responses, n (%)	p-value*
PTSD (Total n=195)		<0.0001
0.0-2.0g	79 (40.51%)	
2.1-4.0g	42 (21.54%)	
4.1-6.0g	19 (9.74%)	
6.1-8.0g	14 (7.18%)	
8.1-10.0g or more	41 (21.03%)	
Non-PTSD (Total n=509)		
0.0-2.0g	356 (69.94%)	
2.1-4.0g	83 (16.31%)	
4.1-6.0g	43 (8.45%)	
6.1-8.0g	18 (3.54%)	
8.1-10.0g or more	9 (1.77%)	

PTSD – Post traumatic stress disorder.
* Bolded p-values are statistically significant.

USAGE OF MEDICAL CANNABIS

Patient reported daily usage of medical cannabis (in grams) is shown in Table 4. At 4 month follow-up, a total of 195 PTSD and 509 non-PTSD patients responded to the question asking them to specify the amount used per day. Significantly more PTSD patients reported taking higher doses than non-PTSD patients (21.03% using 8.1g or more vs. 1.77%, p<0.0001).

DISCUSSION

Different varieties of medical cannabis were reported to be effective for managing PTSD as an overall condition, and for managing common condition-related symptoms, namely depression, anxiety, sleep problems, and pain. Notably, *Sedamen^{MR}* was reported to be beneficial for PTSD after 4 and 10 months, as well as for the four PTSD symptoms most commonly experienced by surveyed patients. Other popular varieties included *Luminarium^{MR}*, which was reported to provide relief from all symptoms except sleep problems, *Midnight^{MR}*, which was effective in managing all symptoms but not the overall condition after only four months, and *Alaska^{MR}*, which was present in the list of effective varieties for all symptoms except pain and PTSD as an overall condition after 10 months. These trends are important to understand when determining which varieties are best suited for patients depending on the symptoms they are experiencing.

The two varieties reported to be most effective for managing PTSD at 4 and at 10 months were *Sedamen^{MR}* and *Luminarium^{MR}*. Interestingly, *Sedamen^{MR}* is an *indica* dominant variety whereas *Luminarium^{MR}* is *sativa* dominant. The THC and CBD contents of the two varieties, however, are similar. It is thought that the *indica/sativa* properties of different cannabis varieties play a role in their physiological effects, so these results may either suggest that patients prefer a combination of the two for the management of PTSD, or that due to the complicated nature of the disease, with varying phenotypically distinct symptoms, different patients have different needs which are reflected in their reported preferences for cannabis varieties.

In addition to identifying preferred varieties, this study also revealed several other important trends. Notably, PTSD patients reported significant improvement compared to deterioration in their condition following the use of medical cannabis ($p=0.0031$). Additionally, significant improvements were observed in all of the common symptoms of PTSD ($p<0.0001$ for all symptoms). These observations suggest that medical cannabis is a highly effective treatment option for PTSD patients, either in addition to or as an alternative to traditional psychotherapy and pharmacotherapy, and should be further investigated in controlled efficacy studies.

Within the limits of what is prescribed by their physicians, many patients self-titrate their dose to be able to optimally manage their symptoms. It was observed in this study that patients with PTSD consume significantly more cannabis than non-PTSD patients (p<0.0001). One explanation for this difference in dosing may be that a large proportion of patients with PTSD in this population are military veterans who receive insurance coverage through Veteran's Affairs Canada for their medication. Because other patient populations do not yet have access to coverage for this medication, cost can be a limiting factor in terms of products selected and amount consumed. This could have contributed to the observation of the higher quantities used and varieties preferred by PTSD patients compared to non-PTSD patients. This factor should be further investigated to give clinicians a better understanding of the optimal daily dose of cannabis that is both safe and efficacious for managing PTSD. Additionally, since patients were often ordering multiple varieties at a time, it is likely that they often medicated with several different strains on a daily basis. This may have made it difficult for them to differentiate which strains were responsible for improvements in particular symptoms, especially if a combination of strains provided a unique cumulative effect. This does not call into question the efficacy of cannabis as a treatment option for PTSD patients, but rather suggests that further research in a controlled clinical setting is needed to provide further insight into the efficacy of individual strains for treating specific symptoms.

CONCLUSION

Several varieties of medical cannabis have been reported by PTSD patients to provide effective relief from their condition and associated symptoms. The most preferred strain for managing PTSD and all related symptoms was *Sedamen^{MR}*. Among respondents at 4 and 10 month follow-up intervals, many also reported *Luminarium^{MR}* to be an effective variety for managing this condition. Additionally, *Midnight^{MR}* was found to be effective in relieving each of the four most common symptoms associated with PTSD (depression, anxiety, sleep problems, and pain). As cannabis becomes a more widely available treatment option for PTSD, this data will become increasingly valuable for helping physicians and patients select varieties that are best suited for them to more quickly and effectively manage the symptoms they are experiencing. In addition, it is important for informing the effective design of controlled efficacy studies that will be conducted in the future to further investigate the clinical utility of medical cannabis in this patient population.

ACKNOWLEDGMENTS

We thank the generous support of Bratty Family Fund, Michael and Karyn Goldstein Cancer Research Fund, Joey and Mary Furfari Cancer Research Fund, Pulenzas Cancer Research Fund, Joseph and Silvana Melara Cancer Research Fund, and Ofelia Cancer Research Fund. This study was conducted in collaboration with MedReleaf.

REFERENCES

[1]   Sherin JE, Nemeroff CB. Post-traumatic stress disorder: the neurobiological impact of psychological trauma. Dialogues Clin Neurosci 2011;13:263-78.

[2]   Greer GR, Grob CS, Halberstadt AL. PTSD symptom reports of patients evaluated for the New Mexico medical cannabis program. J Psychoactive Drugs 2014;46(1):73-7

[3]   Walsh Z, Gonzalez R, Crosby K, Thiessen MS, Carroll C, Bonn-Miller MO. Medical cannabis and mental health: A guided systematic review. Clin Psychol Rev 2017;51:15-29.

[4]   Schmeltzer SN, Herman JP, Sah R. Neuropeptide Y (NPY) and posttraumatic stress disorder (PTSD): A translational update. Exp Neurol 2017;284:196-210.

[5]   Woon FL, Farrer TJ, Braman CR, Mabey JK, Hedges DW. A meta-analysis of the relationship between symptom severity of Posttraumatic Stress Disorder and executive function. CognNeuropsychiatry 2016;22(1):1-16.

[6]   McCarty R. Learning about stress: neural, endocrine and behavioral adaptations. Stress 2016;19(5):449-475.

[7]   Yehuda R. Advances in understanding neuroendocrine alterations in PTSD and their therapeutic implications. Ann NY Acad Sci 2006;1071:137-66.

[8]   Resnick HS, Yehuda R, Pitman RK, Foy DW. Effect of previous trauma on acute plasma cortisol level following rape. Am J Psychiatry1995;152:1675-77.

[9]   Yehuda R, McFarlane AC, Shalev AY. Predicting the development of posttraumatic stress disorder from the acute response to a traumatic event. Biol Psychiatry1998;44:1305-13.

[10]   Wang S, Mason, J. Elevations of serum T3 levels and their association with symptoms in WWII veterans with combat-related posttraumatic stress disorder: replication of findings in Vietnam combat veterans. Psychosom Med 1999;61:131-8.

[11]   Todd SM, Zhou C, Clarke DJ, Chohan TW, Bahceci D, Arnold JC. Interactions between cannabidiol and Δ9-THC following acute and repeated dosing: Rebound hyperactivity, sensorimotor gating and epigenetic and neuroadaptive changes in the mesolimbic pathway. Eur Neuropsychopharmacol 2016 Dec 30.

SECTION TWO: ACKNOWLEDGMENTS

In: Medical Cannabis   ISBN: 978-1-53611-907-7
Editors: S. O'Hearn, A. Blake et al.   © 2017 Nova Science Publishers, Inc.

Chapter 11

ABOUT THE EDITORS

Shannon O'Hearn, BScH, MSc is the Project Manager of Clinical Research at MedReleaf Corp. and is responsible for the oversight of project planning, protocol development, regulatory and ethics submissions, scientific writing, and other research initiatives sponsored by MedReleaf Corp. She completed a Bachelor of Science with honours in Environmental Life Sciences through Queen's University (Kingston, ON) and Trinity College Dublin (Dublin, IE), and following that completed a Master's of Science in Clinical Research Administration through Walden University. Email: SOhearn@medreleaf.com

Alexia Blake, BASc, MSc graduated from the Honours Nanotechnology Engineering program at the University of Waterloo before obtaining a Masters in Food Science from the University of Guelph. In her role as Product Development Engineer at MedReleaf Corp., she oversees all product development initiatives, and works closely with the Clinical Research team to understand the challenges associated with medical cannabis use and identify how these concerns may be resolved by novel or improved cannabis products that offer unique product features related to dosing, efficacy, and method of administration. Email: ABlake@medreleaf.com

Bo Angela Wan, BA, MPhil is a clinical research assistant in the Rapid Response Radiotherapy Program at the Odette Cancer Centre, Sunnybrook Health Sciences Centre, Toronto, Canada, and completed her education at the University of Cambridge in the United Kingdom under the Blyth Cambridge Commonwealth Trust Scholarship. She previously conducted research on the neurobiology of fruit fly olfaction and her current interests lie in cancer bioimarkers and palliative medicine.
Email: Angela.Wan@sunnybrook.ca

Stephanie Chan, BSc(C) is a clinical research assistant in the Rapid Response Radiotherapy Program at the Odette Cancer Centre, Sunnybrook Health Sciences Centre, Toronto, Canada, and also a biochemistry student at the University of Waterloo, Canada. She was the recipient of the J Frank Brookfield Scholarship for excellence in biology and the Don E Irish Scholarship in Science from the University of Waterloo in 2016.
Email: Stephanie.Chan@sunnybrook.ca

Edward Chow, MBBS, MSc, PhD, FRCPC is Professor of Radiation Oncology at the University of Toronto in Canada. He is the chair of the Rapid Response Radiotherapy Program and Bone Metastases Site Group at the Odette Cancer Centre, Sunnybrook Health Scienes Centre, Toronto, Canada, and also a senior scientist at the Sunnybrook Research Institute. He has published in the area of palliative radiotherapy and end of life care issues. Email: Edward.Chow@sunnybrook.ca

Joav Merrick, MD, MMedSci, DMSc, born and educated in Denmark is professor of pediatrics, child health and human development, Division of Pediatrics, Hadassah Hebrew University Medical Center, Mt Scopus Campus, Jerusalem, Israel and Kentucky Children's Hospital, University of Kentucky, Lexington, Kentucky United States and professor of public health at the Center for Healthy Development, School of Public Health, Georgia State University, Atlanta, United States, the medical director of the Health Services, Division for Intellectual and Developmental Disabilities, Ministry of Social Affairs and Social Services, Jerusalem, the

founder and director of the National Institute of Child Health and Human Development in Israel. Numerous publications in the field of pediatrics, child health and human development, rehabilitation, intellectual disability, disability, health, welfare, abuse, advocacy, quality of life and prevention. Received the Peter Sabroe Child Award for outstanding work on behalf of Danish Children in 1985 and the International LEGO-Prize ("The Children's Nobel Prize") for an extraordinary contribution towards improvement in child welfare and well-being in 1987.
Email: jmerrick@zahav.net.il

In: Medical Cannabis   ISBN: 978-1-53611-907-7
Editors: S. O'Hearn, A. Blake et al.   © 2017 Nova Science Publishers, Inc.

Chapter 12

ABOUT THE RAPID RESPONSE RADIOTHERAPY PROGRAM AT THE ODETTE CANCER CENTRE, SUNNYBROOK HEALTH SCIENCES CENTRE, TORONTO, CANADA

The Odette Cancer Centre, the comprehensive cancer program of Sunnybrook Health Sciences Centre is a leading regional cancer centre in Toronto, Ontario, Canada. It is the sixth largest cancer centre in North America in terms of number of new cancer patients seen per year. The Department of Radiation Oncology at Sunnybrook is an academic unit fully affiliated with the University of Toronto. Palliative radiotherapy is one of the key research foci in the Department of Radiation Oncology. The Rapid Response Radiotherapy Program (RRRP) is a specialized clinic designed to provide timely palliative radiotherapy. The RRRP was developed in 1996, and approximately 500-600 patients are seen in one year. This program aims to improve the quality of life of palliative cancer patients, while decreasing wait time and allowing for same day treatment.

Contact

Professor Edward Chow, MBBS, PhD, FRCPC, Department of Radiation Oncology, Odette Cancer Centre, Sunnybrook Health Sciences Centre, 2075 Bayview Avenue, Toronto, Ontario, Canada M4N 3M5.
E-mail: Edward.Chow@sunnybrook.ca

In: Medical Cannabis   ISBN: 978-1-53611-907-7
Editors: S. O'Hearn, A. Blake et al. © 2017 Nova Science Publishers, Inc.

Chapter 13

ABOUT THE NATIONAL INSTITUTE OF CHILD HEALTH AND HUMAN DEVELOPMENT IN ISRAEL

The National Institute of Child Health and Human Development (NICHD) in Israel was established in 1998 as a virtual institute under the auspices of the Medical Director, Ministry of Social Affairs and Social Services in order to function as the research arm for the Office of the Medical Director. In 1998 the National Council for Child Health and Pediatrics, Ministry of Health and in 1999 the Director General and Deputy Director General of the Ministry of Health endorsed the establishment of the NICHD.

Mission

The mission of a National Institute for Child Health and Human Development in Israel is to provide an academic focal point for the scholarly interdisciplinary study of child life, health, public health, welfare, disability, rehabilitation, intellectual disability and related aspects of human development. This mission includes research, teaching, clinical work, information and public service activities in the field of child health and human development.

Service and academic activities

Over the years many activities became focused in the south of Israel due to collaboration with various professionals at the Faculty of Health Sciences (FOHS) at the Ben Gurion University of the Negev (BGU). Since 2000 an affiliation with the Zusman Child Development Center at the Pediatric Division of Soroka University Medical Center has resulted in collaboration around the establishment of the Down Syndrome Clinic at that center. In 2002 a full course on "Disability" was established at the Recanati School for Allied Professions in the Community, FOHS, BGU and in 2005 collaboration was started with the Primary Care Unit of the faculty and disability became part of the master of public health course on "Children and society". In the academic year 2005-2006 a one semester course on "Aging with disability" was started as part of the master of science program in gerontology in our collaboration with the Center for Multidisciplinary Research in Aging. In 2010 collaborations with the Division of Pediatrics, Hadassah Hebrew University Medical Center, Jerusalem, Israel around the National Down Syndrome Center and teaching students and residents about intellectual and developmental disabilities as part of their training at this campus.

Research activities

The affiliated staff have over the years published work from projects and research activities in this national and international collaboration. In the year 2000 the International Journal of Adolescent Medicine and Health and in 2005 the International Journal on Disability and Human Development of De Gruyter Publishing House (Berlin and New York) were affiliated with the National Institute of Child Health and Human Development. From

2008 also the International Journal of Child Health and Human Development (Nova Science, New York), the International Journal of Child and Adolescent Health (Nova Science) and the Journal of Pain Management (Nova Science) affiliated and from 2009 the International Public Health Journal (Nova Science) and Journal of Alternative Medicine Research (Nova Science). All peer-reviewed international journals.

National collaborations

Nationally the NICHD works in collaboration with the Faculty of Health Sciences, Ben Gurion University of the Negev; Department of Physical Therapy, Sackler School of Medicine, Tel Aviv University; Autism Center, Assaf HaRofeh Medical Center; National Rett and PKU Centers at Chaim Sheba Medical Center, Tel HaShomer; Department of Physiotherapy, Haifa University; Department of Education, Bar Ilan University, Ramat Gan, Faculty of Social Sciences and Health Sciences; College of Judea and Samaria in Ariel and in 2011 affiliation with Center for Pediatric Chronic Diseases and National Center for Down Syndrome, Department of Pediatrics, Hadassah Hebrew University Medical Center, Mount Scopus Campus, Jerusalem.

International collaborations

Internationally with the Department of Disability and Human Development, College of Applied Health Sciences, University of Illinois at Chicago; Strong Center for Developmental Disabilities, Golisano Children's Hospital at Strong, University of Rochester School of Medicine and Dentistry, New York; Centre on Intellectual Disabilities, University of Albany, New York; Centre for Chronic Disease Prevention and Control, Health Canada, Ottawa; Chandler Medical Center and Children's Hospital, Kentucky Children's Hospital, Section of Adolescent Medicine, University of Kentucky, Lexington; Chronic Disease Prevention and Control Research

Center, Baylor College of Medicine, Houston, Texas; Division of Neuroscience, Department of Psychiatry, Columbia University, New York; Institute for the Study of Disadvantage and Disability, Atlanta; Center for Autism and Related Disorders, Department Psychiatry, Children's Hospital Boston, Boston; Department of Pediatric and Adolescent Medicine, Western Michigan University Homer Stryker MD School of Medicine, Kalamazoo, Michigan, United States; Department of Paediatrics, Child Health and Adolescent Medicine, Children's Hospital at Westmead, Westmead, Australia; International Centre for the Study of Occupational and Mental Health, Düsseldorf, Germany; Centre for Advanced Studies in Nursing, Department of General Practice and Primary Care, University of Aberdeen, Aberdeen, United Kingdom; Quality of Life Research Center, Copenhagen, Denmark; Nordic School of Public Health, Gottenburg, Sweden, Scandinavian Institute of Quality of Working Life, Oslo, Norway; The Department of Applied Social Sciences (APSS) of The Hong Kong Polytechnic University Hong Kong.

Targets

Our focus is on research, international collaborations, clinical work, teaching and policy in health, disability and human development and to establish the NICHD as a permanent institute in Israel in order to conduct model research and together with the four university schools of public health/medicine in Israel establish a national master and doctoral program in disability and human development at the institute to secure the next generation of professionals working in this often non-prestigious/low-status field of work.

Contact

Joav Merrick, MD, MMedSci, DMSc
Professor of Pediatrics
Medical Director, Health Services, Division for Intellectual and Developmental Disabilities, Ministry of Social Affairs and Social Services, POB 1260, IL-91012 Jerusalem, Israel.
E-mail: jmerrick@zahav.net.il

In: Medical Cannabis   ISBN: 978-1-53611-907-7
Editors: S. O'Hearn, A. Blake et al. © 2017 Nova Science Publishers, Inc.

Chapter 14

ABOUT THE BOOK SERIES "HEALTH AND HUMAN DEVELOPMENT"

Health and human development is a book series with publications from a multidisciplinary group of researchers, practitioners and clinicians for an international professional forum interested in the broad spectrum of health and human development. Books already published:

- Merrick J, Omar HA, eds. Adolescent behavior research. International perspectives. New York: Nova Science, 2007.
- Kratky KW. Complementary medicine systems: Comparison and integration. New York: Nova Science, 2008.
- Schofield P, Merrick J, eds. Pain in children and youth. New York: Nova Science, 2009.
- Greydanus DE, Patel DR, Pratt HD, Calles Jr JL, eds. Behavioral pediatrics, 3 ed. New York: Nova Science, 2009.
- Ventegodt S, Merrick J, eds. Meaningful work: Research in quality of working life. New York: Nova Science, 2009.
- Omar HA, Greydanus DE, Patel DR, Merrick J, eds. Obesity and adolescence. A public health concern. New York: Nova Science, 2009.
- Lieberman A, Merrick J, eds. Poverty and children. A public health concern. New York: Nova Science, 2009.

- Goodbread J. Living on the edge. The mythical, spiritual and philosophical roots of social marginality. New York: Nova Science, 2009.
- Bennett DL, Towns S, Elliot E, Merrick J, eds. Challenges in adolescent health: An Australian perspective. New York: Nova Science, 2009.
- Schofield P, Merrick J, eds. Children and pain. New York: Nova Science, 2009.
- Sher L, Kandel I, Merrick J, eds. Alcohol-related cognitive disorders: Research and clinical perspectives. New York: Nova Science, 2009.
- Anyanwu EC. Advances in environmental health effects of toxigenic mold and mycotoxins. New York: Nova Science, 2009.
- Bell E, Merrick J, eds. Rural child health. International aspects. New York: Nova Science, 2009.
- Dubowitz H, Merrick J, eds. International aspects of child abuse and neglect. New York: Nova Science, 2010.
- Shahtahmasebi S, Berridge D. Conceptualizing behavior: A practical guide to data analysis. New York: Nova Science, 2010.
- Wernik U. Chance action and therapy. The playful way of changing. New York: Nova Science, 2010.
- Omar HA, Greydanus DE, Patel DR, Merrick J, eds. Adolescence and chronic illness. A public health concern. New York: Nova Science, 2010.
- Patel DR, Greydanus DE, Omar HA, Merrick J, eds. Adolescence and sports. New York: Nova Science, 2010.
- Shek DTL, Ma HK, Merrick J, eds. Positive youth development: Evaluation and future directions in a Chinese context. New York: Nova Science, 2010.
- Shek DTL, Ma HK, Merrick J, eds. Positive youth development: Implementation of a youth program in a Chinese context. New York: Nova Science, 2010.
- Omar HA, Greydanus DE, Tsitsika AK, Patel DR, Merrick J, eds. Pediatric and adolescent sexuality and gynecology: Principles for the primary care clinician. New York: Nova Science, 2010.
- Chow E, Merrick J, eds. Advanced cancer. Pain and quality of life. New York: Nova Science, 2010.
- Latzer Y, Merrick, J, Stein D, eds. Understanding eating disorders. Integrating culture, psychology and biology. New York: Nova Science, 2010.

- Sahgal A, Chow E, Merrick J, eds. Bone and brain metastases: Advances in research and treatment. New York: Nova Science, 2010.
- Postolache TT, Merrick J, eds. Environment, mood disorders and suicide. New York: Nova Science, 2010.
- Maharajh HD, Merrick J, eds. Social and cultural psychiatry experience from the Caribbean Region. New York: Nova Science, 2010.
- Mirsky J. Narratives and meanings of migration. New York: Nova Science, 2010.
- Harvey PW. Self-management and the health care consumer. New York: Nova Science, 2011.
- Ventegodt S, Merrick J. Sexology from a holistic point of view. New York: Nova Science, 2011.
- Ventegodt S, Merrick J. Principles of holistic psychiatry: A textbook on holistic medicine for mental disorders. New York: Nova Science, 2011.
- Greydanus DE, Calles Jr JL, Patel DR, Nazeer A, Merrick J, eds. Clinical aspects of psychopharmacology in childhood and adolescence. New York: Nova Science, 2011.
- Bell E, Seidel BM, Merrick J, eds. Climate change and rural child health. New York: Nova Science, 2011.
- Bell E, Zimitat C, Merrick J, eds. Rural medical education: Practical strategies. New York: Nova Science, 2011.
- Latzer Y, Tzischinsky. The dance of sleeping and eating among adolescents: Normal and pathological perspectives. New York: Nova Science, 2011.
- Deshmukh VD. The astonishing brain and holistic consciousness: Neuroscience and Vedanta perspectives. New York: Nova Science, 2011.
- Bell E, Westert GP, Merrick J, eds. Translational research for primary healthcare. New York: Nova Science, 2011.
- Shek DTL, Sun RCF, Merrick J, eds. Drug abuse in Hong Kong: Development and evaluation of a prevention program. New York: Nova Science, 2011.
- Ventegodt S, Hermansen TD, Merrick J. Human Development: Biology from a holistic point of view. New York: Nova Science, 2011.
- Ventegodt S, Merrick J. Our search for meaning in life. New York: Nova Science, 2011.

- Caron RM, Merrick J, eds. Building community capacity: Minority and immigrant populations. New York: Nova Science, 2012.
- Klein H, Merrick J, eds. Human immunodeficiency virus (HIV) research: Social science aspects. New York: Nova Science, 2012.
- Lutzker JR, Merrick J, eds. Applied public health: Examining multifaceted Social or ecological problems and child maltreatment. New York: Nova Science, 2012.
- Chemtob D, Merrick J, eds. AIDS and tuberculosis: Public health aspects. New York: Nova Science, 2012.
- Ventegodt S, Merrick J. Textbook on evidence-based holistic mind-body medicine: Basic principles of healing in traditional Hippocratic medicine. New York: Nova Science, 2012.
- Ventegodt S, Merrick J. Textbook on evidence-based holistic mind-body medicine: Holistic practice of traditional Hippocratic medicine. New York: Nova Science, 2012.
- Ventegodt S, Merrick J. Textbook on evidence-based holistic mind-body medicine: Healing the mind in traditional Hippocratic medicine. New York: Nova Science, 2012.
- Ventegodt S, Merrick J. Textbook on evidence-based holistic mind-body medicine: Sexology and traditional Hippocratic medicine. New York: Nova Science, 2012.
- Ventegodt S, Merrick J. Textbook on evidence-based holistic mind-body medicine: Research, philosophy, economy and politics of traditional Hippocratic medicine. New York: Nova Science, 2012.
- Caron RM, Merrick J, eds. Building community capacity: Skills and principles. New York: Nova Science, 2012.
- Lemal M, Merrick J, eds. Health risk communication. New York: Nova Science, 2012.
- Ventegodt S, Merrick J. Textbook on evidence-based holistic mind-body medicine: Basic philosophy and ethics of traditional Hippocratic medicine. New York: Nova Science, 2013.
- Caron RM, Merrick J, eds. Building community capacity: Case examples from around the world. New York: Nova Science, 2013.
- Steele RE. Managed care in a public setting. New York: Nova Science, 2013.
- Srabstein JC, Merrick J, eds. Bullying: A public health concern. New York: Nova Science, 2013.
- Pulenzas N, Lechner B, Thavarajah N, Chow E, Merrick J, eds. Advanced cancer: Managing symptoms and quality of life. New York: Nova Science, 2013.

- Stein D, Latzer Y, eds. Treatment and recovery of eating disorders. New York: Nova Science, 2013.
- Sun J, Buys N, Merrick J. Health promotion: Community singing as a vehicle to promote health. New York: Nova Science, 2013.
- Pulenzas N, Lechner B, Thavarajah N, Chow E, Merrick J, eds. Advanced cancer: Managing symptoms and quality of life. New York: Nova Science, 2013.
- Sun J, Buys N, Merrick J. Health promotion: Strengthening positive health and preventing disease. New York: Nova Science, 2013.
- Merrick J, Israeli S, eds. Food, nutrition and eating behavior. New York: Nova Science, 2013.
- Shahtahmasebi S, Merrick J. Suicide from a public health perspective. New York: Nova Science, 2014.
- Merrick J, Tenenbaum A, eds. Public health concern: Smoking, alcohol and substance use. New York: Nova Science, 2014.
- Merrick J, Aspler S, Morad M, eds. Mental health from an international perspective. New York: Nova Science, 2014.
- Merrick J, ed. India: Health and human development aspects. New York: Nova Science, 2014.
- Caron R, Merrick J, eds. Public health: Improving health via inter-professional collaborations. New York: Nova Science, 2014.
- Merrick J, ed. Pain Mangement Yearbook 2014. New York: Nova Science, 2015.
- Merrick J, ed. Public Health Yearbook 2014. New York: Nova Science, 2015.
- Sher L, Merrick J, eds. Forensic psychiatry: A public health perspective. New York: Nova Science, 2015.
- Shek DTL, Wu FKY, Merrick J, eds. Leadership and service learning education: Holistic development for Chinese university students. New York: Nova Science, 2015.
- Calles JL, Greydanus DE, Merrick J, eds. Mental and holistic health: Some international perspectives. New York: Nova Science, 2015.
- Lechner B, Chow R, Pulenzas N, Popovic M, Zhang N, Zhang X, Chow E, Merrick J, eds. Cancer: Treatment, decision making and quality of life. New York: Nova Science, 2016.
- Lechner B, Chow R, Pulenzas N, Popovic M, Zhang N, Zhang X, Chow E, Merrick J, eds. Cancer: Pain and symptom management. New York: Nova Science, 2016.

- Lechner B, Chow R, Pulenzas N, Popovic M, Zhang N, Zhang X, Chow E, Merrick J, eds. Cancer: Bone metastases, CNS metastases and pathological fractures. New York: Nova Science, 2016.
- Lechner B, Chow R, Pulenzas N, Popovic M, Zhang N, Zhang X, Chow E, Merrick J, eds. Cancer: Spinal cord, lung, breast, cervical, prostate, head and neck cancer. New York: Nova Science, 2016.
- Lechner B, Chow R, Pulenzas N, Popovic M, Zhang N, Zhang X, Chow E, Merrick J, eds. Cancer: Survival, quality of life and ethical implications. New York: Nova Science, 2016.
- Davidovitch N, Gross Z, Ribakov Y, Slobodianiuk A, eds. Quality, mobility and globalization in the higher education system: A comparative look at the challenges of academic teaching. New York: Nova Science, 2016.
- Henry B, Agarwal A, Chow E, Omar HA, Merrick J, eds. Cannabis: Medical aspects. New York: Nova Science, 2017.
- Henry B, Agarwal A, Chow E, Merrick J, eds. Palliative care: Psychosocial and ethical considerations. New York: Nova Science, 2017.
- Furfari A, Charames GS, McDonald R, Rowbottom L, Azad A, Chan S, Wan BA, Chow R, DeAngelis C, Zaki P, Chow E, Merrick J, eds. Oncology: The promising future of biomarkers. New York: Nova Science, 2017.

Contact

Professor Joav Merrick, MD, MMedSci, DMSc
Medical Director, Health Services
Division for Intellectual and Developmental Disabilities
Ministry of Social Affairs and Social Services
POBox 1260, IL-91012 Jerusalem, Israel
E-mail: jmerrick@zahav.net.il

SECTION THREE: INDEX

INDEX

post-traumatic stress disorder (PTSD), 4,
18, 22, 23, 26, 35, 44, 45, 46, 47, 58, 61,
62, 63, 64, 71, 85, 87, 90, 95, 96, 97, 98,
99, 100, 101, 102, 106, 108, 109, 110,
111, 112, 113, 115, 116, 117, 118, 119,
120, 123, 124, 125, 126, 127, 128, 129,
130, 133, 134, 135, 136, 137, 138,
139,141, 142, 143, 144, 145, 147, 148,
149, 150, 151, 152, 153, 154, 155, 156,
157, 158, 159
primary cancers, 44
principal component analysis, 26, 27
products, 5, 6, 82, 127, 158
progestin, 53
prolonged exposure therapy, 97
prostate, 40, 44, 46, 180
psychoactive effects, 40, 41, 49, 52, 68, 70,
71, 72, 108, 109, 126
psychotherapy, 116, 117, 118, 128, 134,
136, 137, 139, 142, 143, 144, 148, 149,
157

Q

quality of life, 14, 23, 26, 27, 35, 36, 37, 40,
49, 50, 51, 58, 60, 66, 67, 69, 80, 83, 88,
93, 96, 99, 100, 104, 105, 113, 116, 118,
130, 135, 150, 151, 165, 167, 176, 178,
179, 180

R

randomized control trial, 52, 71
re-experiencing, 96, 116, 135, 142, 148
research, 4, 5, 7, 11, 22, 25, 26, 34, 35, 36,
41, 55, 73, 76, 79, 92, 111, 129, 136,
142, 143, 144, 147, 148, 158, 159, 163,
164, 167, 169, 170, 171, 172, 175, 176,
177, 178
route of administration, 81

S

safety, 5, 55, 58, 77, 109, 111, 128, 130
sativa, 12, 41, 80, 82, 84, 86, 87, 121, 140,
149, 153, 154, 155, 157
scientific, 4, 5, 7, 14, 41, 59, 82, 83, 92, 99,
163
selective serotonin reuptake inhibitor(s)
(SSRIs), 97, 117, 136
sex, 14, 15, 16, 42, 60, 99, 138
sexual function, 15, 43, 49, 51, 60, 68, 70,
80, 84, 88, 89, 100, 104, 106
side effects, 40, 41, 43, 49, 52, 55, 58, 61,
68, 70, 71, 72, 73, 96, 100, 108, 109, 128
sleep, 12, 13, 15, 18, 19, 20, 21, 22, 26, 28,
30, 31, 32, 34, 35, 36, 37, 40, 41, 43, 44,
45, 47, 48, 49, 51, 54, 55, 58, 60, 61, 62,
63, 64, 65, 66, 68, 69, 71, 72, 74, 75, 80,
81, 84, 85, 87, 88, 90, 96, 97, 100, 101,
102, 104, 106, 107, 109, 120, 126, 127,
148, 151, 152, 153, 154, 155, 156, 158
sleep disorder(s), 12, 18, 20, 21, 22, 26, 35,
44, 45, 47, 58, 61, 62, 63, 64, 71, 75, 85,
87, 90, 101, 102, 104
sleep interference, 26, 28, 30, 31, 32, 34, 36
sleep problems, 12, 19, 20, 21, 40, 48, 63,
65, 66, 74, 85, 87, 88, 90, 106, 107, 148,
151, 152, 153, 154, 155, 156, 158
sleepiness, 40, 49, 52, 68, 70, 71, 108, 109
spasticity, 73, 81
strain, 5, 6, 7, 26, 36, 80, 82, 86, 89, 90, 91,
92, 122, 137, 153, 158
stress, 4, 18, 22, 23, 26, 35, 44, 45, 46, 47,
58, 61, 62, 63, 64, 71, 85, 87, 90, 95, 96,
97, 98, 99, 100, 101, 102, 106, 108, 109,
110, 111, 112, 113, 115, 116, 117, 118,
119, 120, 123, 124, 125, 126, 127, 128,
129, 130, 133, 134, 135, 136, 137, 138,
139,141, 142, 143, 144, 145, 147, 148,
149, 150, 151, 152, 153, 154, 155, 156,
157, 158, 159

T

V

W